PAIN IN PRACTICE

Theory and Treatment Strategies for Manual Therapists

For Butterworth-Heinemann:

Senior Commissioning Editor: Heidi Harrison
Development Editor: Siobhan Campbell
Production Manager: Nancy Arnott
Design: Andy Chapman

PAIN IN PRACTICE

Theory and Treatment Strategies for Manual Therapists

Hubert van Griensven MSc(Pain) BSc DipAc
Consultant Physiotherapist, Southend Hospital NHS Trust, Essex

Foreword by
Douglas Justins
Consultant in Pain Management and Anaesthesia, Pain Management Centre, St Thomas' Hospital, London

With contributions from
Sarah Barker BSc(Hons) PhD(Clin Psych)
Clinical Psychologist, Pain Management Centre, St Thomas' Hospital, London

Helen Galindo, BSc
Physiotherapist, Flinders Medical Centre, Adelaide

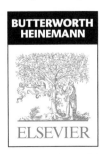

BUTTERWORTH
HEINEMANN

ELSEVIER

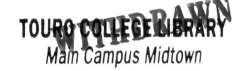
EDINBURGH LONDON NEW YORK OXFORD PHILADELPHIA ST LOUIS SYDNEY TORONTO 2005

This book represents a timely, brave and challenging departure from the purely physical, mechanistic approaches that are so often based on reductionist, single-causation explanations. It attempts to provide an integrated neurophysiological basis for the wide variety of techniques used by manual therapists. There is repeated emphasises that any presumed site of injury has to be analysed in the context of the whole individual who possesses, amongst other things, a dynamic nervous system and a very complex brain.

Rehabilitation and return to normal function are the prime objectives for many patients with pain and it is now realised that many therapies or interventions are merely acting to facilitate that process rather than being some sort of miracle cure in themselves. This shift in role is another big challenge for practitioners locked into the biomedical model. Practitioners and therapists of every hue need to analyse what they do and they must not assume that the outcome of any ministration is necessarily a direct consequence of their intervention.

This book is one step along the way to having everyone in the multidisciplinary team speaking the same language when talking about pain. It will lead to improved understanding of the mechanisms of pain which, in turn, will lead to improved pain management for patients and that, after all, is the most desirable and best possible outcome.

Dr Douglas Justins   2005

Acknowledgements

I would like to thank the following people for their contribution to this book. When I was a student, Nol Bernards, Henk van Zutphen and Gert-Jan Raats ignited my interest in the neural basis of physiotherapy. Without their enthusiasm and guidance, this book would never have been written.

The pain team of St Thomas' fuelled my interest further and helped me to develop it into my speciality. In particular, I would like to thank Dr Douglas Justins, Dr Charles Pither, Dr John Wedley, Specialist Nurses Fran Miller and Karen Sanderson, and Vicky Harding for their help in the early days.

Liz Jones has been there all along.

Christine Marryat provided first-hand accounts of James Cyriax and the history of diagnosis in physiotherapy. She has also been an inspiration.

Many colleagues have provided material by sharing their experiences with me. Sarah Barker and Helen Galindo have enriched this book with their chapters. Elsevier Ltd have provided editorial support.

Nikki Petty gave me a chance to start sharing my ideas. She has also provided me with insight and vital reassurance regarding the processes of writing and publishing. Chris Murphy read the first two drafts ot this book. His suggestions and his friendship have been invaluable.

Sarah Jane Ryan also agreed to read the manuscript and give an objective analysis. John Annan has shared ever-broadening horizons with me. He has been a reminder that it is important to look beyond convention and conformism.

Douglas Justins kindly agreed to write the foreword for this text.

Introduction

The old man ruminates for a while. 'It's on the other side of the river.'
He says that he has just come from that side of the river. Can he have
taken the wrong road? The old man cocks an eyebrow and says, 'The
road is not wrong, it is the traveller who is wrong.'

GAO XINGJIAN, SOUL MOUNTAIN

THE DEVELOPMENT OF MANUAL DIAGNOSIS

Manual therapies have a long history [1] and may well be as old as mankind itself. However, the accurate diagnosis of musculoskeletal pathology is a more recent development. Before the advance of diagnostic technology, doctors had to rely on visual inspection and palpation to reach a diagnosis. The definitive confirmation could only come from surgery or post mortem examination, when the tissues thought to be at fault could be subjected to visual inspection.

If a patient presented with pain in a certain part of the body, it would seem reasonable for a surgeon to assume that pathology is present in that area. If pathology was found during subsequent surgery, this could be thought of as confirmatory. However, reality is more complex. For example, if a patient presented with anterior knee pain a surgeon might convince himself that the pain was caused by the patella and operate. If he would find degenerative changes of the patella, he could interpret these findings as confirmation that knee pathology was causing the pain. Treatment following from the diagnosis could consist of immobilization, excision or even amputation.[2]

Unfortunately the link between pathology and pain is tenuous and many patients had surgery that did not address their problem. It took some time before it became clear that pathology of the hip could manifest as anterior thigh and knee pain.[3] Because of this phenomenon of *referred pain*, the degenerative changes in some patient's knees may have been additional rather than primary. Therefore, visual confirmation of the hypothesis did not necessarily constitute definitive evidence.

To confound diagnosis even further, the invasion of the knee by surgical instruments became a new source of pain for some patients. The surgeon had created a self-fulfilling prophecy.

Dr James Cyriax describes how diagnosis was relatively straight-forward in those with bony changes that revealed themselves on radiographs.[4] However, the majority of patients presented with normal X-rays and their diagnosis and treatment were not based on clear principles. Cyriax came to the conclusion that much of their pain had to stem from the soft tissues, which are not seen on X-ray. He resolved to devise a method to diagnose soft tissue pathology. This method was based on the principle of selective tissue tensioning and followed from the observation that the application of pressure and stretch to an inflamed or damaged soft tissue structure elicits pain. In Cyriax' view, the clinician who knew which musculoskeletal structures were stressed by each active, passive and resisted test was in a position to reach a tissue diagnosis. This approach introduced clinical reasoning into the field of physical therapy. Cyriax advocated treatment by manual techniques and injection, undoubtedly saving many from surgery and iatrogenesis. Unfortunately, in doing so he also perpetuated the idea that pain had to be caused by the tissues.

Since Cyriax, other practitioners have developed more techniques for examination and treatment based on their own observations and interpretations. Robin McKenzie adopted his preoccupation with the spinal disc as a source of back pain, but took the concept much further. Geoffrey Maitland introduced a wider array of treatment techniques by systematically integrating constant reassessment with treatment, thereby verifying one's clinical reasoning at every step.[5] He urged therapists to listen to their patients in order to make subjective and objective features fit into a diagnostic picture. Brian Edwards refined the selective tissue-tensioning model for detailed analysis of the apophyseal joints.[6] Vladimir Janda developed the concept that imbalance in the actions of muscle groups could be the cause of poor posture and abnormal movement.[7] He felt that incorrect use of the body caused excessive load bearing forces on certain musculoskeletal structures, resulting in pain. This approach widened the diagnostic picture by investigating coordination and muscle control. Diagnosis was more than the identification of a tissue at fault. It had to include factors that might have caused and perpetuated the pathology.

Overall manual therapy has become increasingly precise and sophisticated. Experienced clinicians can reach impressive diagnoses that are highly specific: a small deep muscle that is not activated at the right moment, the exact portion of a ligament that creates a dysfunction, the headache that ultimately stems from a biomechanical problem in the foot. Many utilize the results of X-rays, MRI scans and other tests. The pervasive underlying belief is that if the manual therapist gains enough skills and knowledge and if tests become precise enough, eventually all musculoskeletal impairments will be diagnosable.

However, despite ongoing efforts a failsafe method for the diagnosis and treatment of musculoskeletal pain has yet to be developed. In an attempt to find the 'tissue at fault', some clinicians have directed their diagnostic gaze to non-musculoskeletal soft tissues, frequently relying to some extent on selective tissue tensioning principles. Robert Elvey and David Butler have highlighted that nerves are connective tissue structures that are subject to mechanical forces.[8] They have introduced mechanical methods of examining and treating the peripheral nervous system and spinal cord, in addition to the traditional neurological investigations. (In fairness, with admirable and rare honesty Butler has recently acknowledged that the mechanical model does not adequately explain pain.) Jean-Pierre Barral has developed the concept that the viscera are suspended from and have mechanical interfaces with musculoskeletal structures.[9] In his model, pain can be caused by mechanical restrictions imposed on the internal organs and treatment is aimed at the restoration of visceral mobility. Craniosacral therapists like W. Sutherland and John Upledger have asserted that cerebrospinal fluid exerts a rhythmic force on the cranial bones.[10,11] A restriction of the mobility of those bones is thought to affect this rhythm, which is allegedly important for mental, emotional and physical wellbeing. Treatment therefore involves subtle correction of the mobility of the cranial bones.

The wish to improve outcomes and explore new methods have been identified as reasons for the ever-increasing range of interventions.[12] Self-doubt resulting from treatment failure drives therapists to learn more techniques and look at ever more obscure types of impairment, in the hope that one day they will be able to deal with most of their patients' problems.

Patients with disabilities and disability experts object to the application of this biomedical model.[13] They argue that it erroneously interprets disabilities as based within the individual, temporary and in need of a cure.[14] To them, biomedical diagnosis is not the Holy Grail. Many disabilities are permanent and cannot be cured. The clinician who tries to impose the biomedical model on every patient with disabilities is likely to get frustrated and the person visiting them is unlikely to be helped.

Like disabilities, persistent pain often exists in absence of an impairment[15] and may therefore be beyond the reach of interventionist treatment. Many patients with genuine pain have all the necessary investigations without ever being diagnosed with an identifiable lesion. Others are given a diagnosis that does not have a cure attached to it, such as an osteoporotic fracture of a vertebral body. The diagnosis is clear, but it does not help them. Both groups of patients may well end up extremely frustrated with the health care professions and vice versa.[16] Both patients and clinicians can benefit from a different approach.

COGNITIVE-BEHAVIOURAL PAIN MANAGEMENT

The way people respond to pain and injury is highly individual. Some remain cheerful and continue to work and go out despite ongoing difficulties. Others suffer immensely, feel unable to do anything and become increasingly disabled. What distinguishes the two may not be the level of pain or the extent of the injury (if present), but a number of psychological and social factors.[12] For example, an important factor is the individual's interpretation of what a pain indicates. Does it mean something is damaged? Can it be ignored or does it require action? Are work and other activities to be avoided or can they be continued. Are the rewards from disability benefit and people taking care of the patient greater than those from labour? Although these issues determine the perception and impact of pain to a great extent, they do not form an integral part of manual therapy.

Many studies have confirmed the effect of psychosocial factors. A well-known example is a 4-year study of a large group of industrial workers.[17,18] All participants were assessed for physical, psychological and workplace factors at the start of the study. Those who developed back pain during the study were no different from those who did not in terms of biomechanics and workplace factors, but they tended to have lower levels of job satisfaction and certain personality traits. The result of another study suggested that fear of what might happen if work was resumed was the best predictor of the length of time off work after back injury.[19]

The factors that determine the individual's pain experience and the negative effect that pain has on their wellbeing, the people around them and their activities, can be addressed in a multidisciplinary Pain Management Programme (PMP). This type of programme aims to give people a realistic understanding of what their pain does and does not mean, and teach them ways of being as active as possible.[20] It reduces the negative impact of pain in a variety of ways. Improving physical fitness, reducing the intake of drugs with unhelpful side-effects and addressing issues related with family and work are some of the ways employed to achieve this.

Typically, a patient must have exhausted all other therapeutic options before they can be accepted for a PMP. It is also important that they have been thoroughly investigated, so that worries about underlying pathologies can be laid to rest. The patient has to come to accept that the medical profession has nothing more to offer, in order for them to take control and address unhelpful beliefs and behaviours. Many patients attending PMPs benefit enormously,[21] learning ways of returning to activities that are important to them and becoming less dependent on medication and other people. Some explore new directions in terms of employment and life fulfilment. These changes can have a positive effect on the perception of pain.

The cognitive-behavioural approach offered by PMPs seems diametrically opposed to hands-on therapy. The patient is discouraged from exploring further clinical diagnosis and treatment, which form the very essence of the biomedical paradigm. The assessment concentrates on levels of function, coping strategies, and social and psychological factors, but does not involve diagnostics. The patient is coached, not treated. He gets explanations, advice, counselling and exercises, but no passive intervention (i.e. intervention in which the patient is passive) is offered. Whereas the manual therapist frequently asks where the pain is and how it has changed, the focus in the pain management approach is on function: how much further can you walk; can you sit for long enough to attend the university course you want to do; are you able to devise strategies to keep working without taking time off sick?

Increasing numbers of clinicians working in private practice and outpatient clinics are aware of the benefits of the hands-off, cognitive-behavioural approach. However, they work in a setting that is very different from the PMP. They are therefore faced with the dilemma of having to choose between two models of clinical reasoning that seem to be mutually exclusive. Figure 1.1 illustrates this. The traditional musculoskeletal model with the arthrokinetic unit at its centre is highly analytical where musculoskeletal structures are concerned. It acknowledges that psychological, nutritional and other factors influence this unit, but these factors are seen as supplementary. In the biopsychosocial model this tissue analysis has all but disappeared. Instead, a host of factors surrounding and influencing the dysfunction and the pain are the focus. Beliefs, coping strategies and fitness are the subjects of analysis. Because each model is poorly represented in the other, it is difficult for therapists to integrate them.

The division of approaches to pain management into two separate camps is highly unsatisfactory for patients. Although some may well

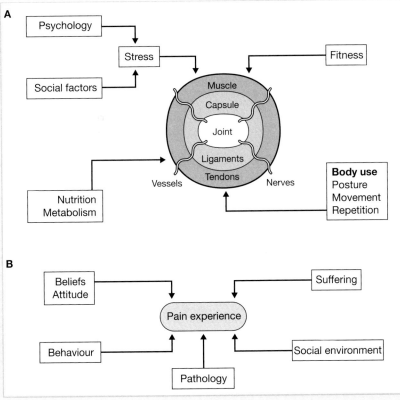

Fig. 1.1 Diagrams representing two conceptual models of musculoskeletal pain. **A.** The traditional musculoskeletal model is based on the arthrokinetic unit of joint and surrounding structures. The factors influencing this unit are of secondary importance. **B.** The biopsychosocial model acknowledges that pain may have a physical component, but focuses on psychological and social influences.

require either one approach or the other, most would benefit from an appropriate selection from each. A patient who is anxious about their pain should not necessarily be excluded from manual treatment, just like the presence of identifiable pathology does not rule out the biopsychosocial model as a viable treatment option.

It is not just the patient who loses out because of the divide in the therapeutic community. Highly successful hands-on clinicians are understandably reluctant to abandon their skills in favour of an approach that does not allow them to 'do something' for, or to, their patients. Those who try to add cognitive-behavioural methods to their treatment arsenal often start with the physical therapy approach they are most familiar with. If the patient fails to respond, they begin all over again, reassessing the patient and this time interpreting their problems using a cognitive-behavioural frame of reference.

This split in clinical reasoning models is frustrating and time consuming. By the time the mechanical model is abandoned both patient and therapist are likely to have lost enthusiasm. As a consequence, the new approach is likely to feel like a compromise and to lose much of its powerful potential. It is not surprising that a US study found that 96% of physiotherapists preferred not to work with patients with chronic pain.[22] In stark contrast is the fact that several epidemiological studies have demonstrated that between 12 and 55% of the general population in the western world suffer with chronic pain.[23] This discrepancy is unacceptable.

AN INTEGRATIVE MODEL FOR THE TREATMENT OF PAIN

Pain is prevalent and therapists are frustrated with their treatment options. The addition of a new treatment paradigm, such as the biopsychosocial model, brings alternatives but seems to force the clinician to abandon the approach they are familiar with. However, many patients require both approaches and it is often not appropriate to choose only one. This book recognizes that there is a need for a unified clinical reasoning model, applicable to every patient complaining of pain. It is important that each patient receives help with the appropriate selection of strategies and techniques.

Both the mechanical musculoskeletal and the cognitive-behavioural approach have an element that is essential for their efficacy but is rarely part of their analysis. It is essential to identify this element, because these two paradigms can only be combined successfully by focusing on what they have in common rather than on what differentiates them. This unifying element is the nervous system that processes pain and responds to pain. Pain arises within the nervous system and without it pain is inconceivable. As researcher and clinician Lorimer Moseley summarizes in his lectures: 'No brain, no pain'. The importance of this simple fact has been recognized by some therapists, but is frequently ignored.[24]

Until the 1960s, the nervous system was thought to passively detect and respond to events in the body. It is now clear that in reality it is highly adaptive. It can amplify or suppress sensations selectively, depending on the importance for the organism as a whole (Box 1.1). It can 'rewire' itself, forming new connections and changing the way pain is perceived in a more permanent way. Under certain circumstances, the nervous system may generate pain without any stimulation at all.

A treatment or action can alter the perception of pain *only* if it affects the activity in the nervous system in some way. If the pain is caused by tissue damage and inflammation the most appropriate treatment is obvious: any intervention that reduces the inflammation and aids the repair of the damaged tissues can inhibit the stimulation of local 'pain nerves' and will therefore be helpful. However, many ongoing pains do not originate in the tissues, but merely manifest there. For example, modern research suggests that pain syndromes seemingly stemming from musculoskeletal structures may be the result of minor neuropathies (an excellent example of this type of research is the work by Greening, Lynn and Leary [25,26]). Unless a therapist is aware of this and uses specific tests to assess function of the peripheral nervous system, signs and symptoms are likely to be misinterpreted and therefore mistreated.

The diagnostic process can be further complicated by the fact that the central nervous system can actively distort perception of pain. As in the first scenario in Box 1.1, the brain decides what needs to be amplified and what can safely be suppressed. This applies to any form of sensory input including pain. The brain's decision about which impulses can be suppressed is not necessarily the most helpful one, as anyone who has walked into a lamppost whilst eyeing an attractive passer-by can appreciate! Similarly, the active intensification of the perception of pain is not always helpful, but sometimes the brain decides to maximize its input for the purpose of analysis. The clinician who understands that sensation is actively modified will assess the way the central nervous system of a patient deals with pain and will involve it in the treatment. A therapy that targets the origin of the pain while also addressing the way pain is being processed has a greater chance of success.

In some patients it is the brain rather than an ongoing tissue dysfunction that maintains the pain. For them, the ongoing search for an effective manual technique is counterproductive. Patients with persistent pain frequently demonstrate an abundance of tender or sore tissues, but these are not necessarily the cause of the pain. The therapist may discover that 'If you look, you will find'.[27] The challenge is therefore not just to find things to treat, but also to determine which findings are relevant. This is highlighted by the fact that lumbar magnetic resonance imaging (MRI) scans are often abnormal in asymptomatic subjects.[28]

The nervous system is equally important for the understanding of the effect of psychosocial interventions on pain. The mind is not a thing on its own, but it has physical correlates in the brain. As far as we know, awareness arises in the brain. Unless cognitive-behavioural

Box 1.1 Examples of how the nervous system controls its own input by enhancing, suppressing or otherwise modifying sensations including pain

Scenario 1. Imagine that you are in a crowded bar. Groups of people around you are talking and laughing. The PA is pumping out the latest rap music. Suddenly you realize that someone sitting at a table a few metres away has mentioned your name and is laughing out loud. Suddenly you no longer hear any of the noise around you, but your ears suck up every word from that table.

Scenario 2. You have just sprained your ankle stepping off the pavement. It hurts and makes you limp. You come to the next pedestrian crossing whilst ruminating about the way this injury may stop you going out in the evening. A loud blast from a horn gives you a start and you see a bus driving straight at you. You sprint to get out of its path. You do not feel your ankle pain until you sit down to catch your breath.

methods affect the way the brain processes pain, they cannot be effective. There is an abundance of evidence for the ways in which mental and emotional states trigger mechanisms in the brain and spinal cord, leading to either suppression or amplification of pain signals. These responses are highly selective, enabling the brain to choose what it perceives. An understanding of the function of the sensory system enables the clinician to maximize its effects in the treatment of pain.

ABOUT THIS BOOK

This book aims to give a clear understanding of the generation of pain and how pain is processed by the nervous system. The physiology and neuroscience behind various pain mechanisms is discussed. It is made clear how pain mechanisms manifest in the descriptions the patient gives and the signs found by the therapist. The differentiation between pain that originates in the tissues and pain that *merely manifests there* forms an important part of the diagnostic process. Recommendations are made for the most appropriate management strategies.

It can be difficult to see how pain science, typically expressed in the reductionist language of neurophysiology and operating on a subcellular level, translates to the more holistic level of the patient. Where possible, this book presents clinical reasoning models that are easily applied in clinical practice. Lecturers and students may be interested in the practical experiments described throughout the text.

There are two principles that run like a thread through every chapter of this book. The most important principle is that the brain is central in the perception of and the response to pain. It constantly analyses input from the body and regulates everything in the body, affecting change through the nervous and endocrine systems. In addition, it interacts with the environment by changing behaviour. The more the brain and therefore these regulating systems are included in our clinical reasoning models, the better the chances of therapeutic success. Every therapeutic encounter provides the patient with a barrage of sensory input, which generates changes in output in terms of motor, autonomic and hormonal activity (Fig. 1.2). Interpreting all our

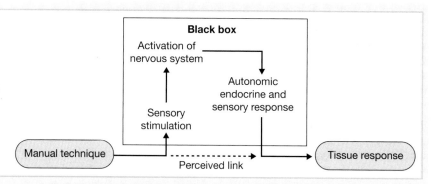

Fig. 1.2 The patient's regulatory systems form a black box. Processes inside the black box are not seen directly. A therapist provides sensory and mechanical input and observes a reaction. The reaction can be interpreted as mechanical, while in reality it relies on subsystems in the black box.

observations and the patient's reports as purely mechanical is irrational and unhelpful.

The second principle is that our analytic process and treatment design need to work from general to specific, especially when it comes to treating patients with ongoing pain. Even when a localized dysfunction is the focus of the visible treatment, the covert clinical reasoning process needs to assign first place to general issues. The traditional musculoskeletal approach tends to treat the lesion first and integrate the use of the recovering structure into the function of the body part next. Finally, function of the body as a whole is addressed if required. This book advocates an approach used by clinicians working with neurological patients, assessing and where necessary addressing general issues before turning to specific impairments. These general issues can be of a psychological or social nature, or they may have to do with the central nervous system or the physiology of stress.

It is the author's experience that once these principles are understood they apply equally well in the acute setting, thereby removing the need for separate approaches for acute and chronic patients. Some readers may feel that they are complicating matters by taking on yet another clinical reasoning model, but the opposite is true. The knowledge and methods presented in this book unify and simplify the vast arsenal of disparate techniques currently used by physical therapists. To paraphrase one of my Chinese internal arts teachers: 'Our practice is really very simple. However, years of dedicated study and practice are required to actually *make* it simple'.

To a large extent, the structure of this book follows the hierarchy present in the nervous system. Chapter 2 describes the perception of stimuli applied to the somatic tissues. Tissue damage, inflammation and repair and the resultant pain are discussed, to give the reader an understanding of 'normal' pain that can be expected to respond to physical treatment. The results of damage to the peripheral nerves and incomplete regeneration are the subject of Chapter 3. This includes subjects such as post-surgical pain and neuralgia, which may masquerade as musculoskeletal or visceral pains.

Impulses from the periphery enter the central nervous system in the dorsal horn, where a process of integration and modification takes place. Chapter 4 deals with the function of this important centre and how it influences the way stimuli are perceived.

Chapter 5 discusses the parts of the autonomic nervous system and the endocrine system that are most relevant for physical therapists. The effects of these systems can make or break any treatment by influencing the healing response. They are regulated both by physical demand and emotional status and are part of the stress response. Complex Regional Pain Syndrome is included because of its apparent autonomic presentation.

I am grateful for Sarah Barker's exposition of psychosocial issues in Chapter 6. I frequently hear the comment from colleagues that they don't want to become psychologists. Sarah's chapter describes psychological issues related to persistent pain, points out when to refer to a clinical psychologist and advises how to discuss this with the patient.

Chapter 7 looks at the role of the brain in the perception and regulation of pain. This is a highly complicated area, so an attempt has been made to limit the material to models and discoveries that can be seen and applied in clinical practice. Links are made between the psychological processes described in Chapter 6 and changes in the way the nervous system deals with pain from Chapter 4.

In clinical practice, assessment of pain and its impact tends to rely on self-reporting and the therapist's subjective judgement. The use of pain scales has been widely publicized and is therefore not discussed specifically in this book. However, few texts provide the clinician with detailed advice on the measurement of function, which is essential for the assessment of the impact of pain and the effectiveness of treatment. I am obliged to Helen Galindo for Chapter 8, which contains detailed inventory and discussion of functional testing outcome measures.

The final chapter brings the material from the whole book together under an overarching model. General principles of assessment and treatment selection are discussed. The elements of the examination process are placed within the context of the nervous system's processing of and response to pain.

A glossary of pain terminology is given in Appendix 1. Appendix 7 has a list of useful websites and addresses.

Patients with persistent pain demand an attitude that combines two seemingly opposing elements. On the one hand, it is important that the clinician is methodical, consistent and reliable. On the other, willingness to take into account the wider impact of pain and to explore new paradigms are required, because a strict and unyielding medical model is often not helpful. In order to stimulate lateral thinking, each chapter starts with a quote that relates to an important element of the text in an oblique way.

Note: the terms manual therapist, therapist, clinician and physical therapist are used interchangeably in this text. In a narrow sense they refer to physiotherapists, physical therapists, osteopaths and chiropractors, but they are by no means restricted to those practitioners.

Reference to gender is avoided as much as possible. Where this is not possible, the male form tends to be used. This is not intended to be derogatory towards women and neither does it indicate that the text applies to men only.

References

[1] Harris J. History and development of manipulation and mobilization. In: Basmajian J, Nyberg R, eds. Rational Manual Therapies. Baltimore: Williams and Wilkins, 1993: 7–19

[2] Bourdillon J. Introduction. Spinal manipulation. London: William Heinemann Medical Books, 1973: 1–13

[3] Winkel D, Fisher S, Vroege C. Weke delen aandoeningen van het bewegingsapparaat (Soft tissue pathology of the musculoskeletal

system). Deel 2: Diagnostiek. Utrecht: Bohn, Scheltema and Holkema, 1984

[4] Cyriax J. Preface. Textbook of orthopaedic medicine. Diagnosis of soft tissue lesions. London: Baillière Tindall, 1982: ix–xi

[5] Maitland G. Vertebral manipulation, 5th edn. London: Butterworths, 1986

[6] Edwards B. Manual of combined movements. Edinburgh: Churchill Livingstone, 1992

[7] Bosman W, Hagenaars L. Kinesiologie. Onderzoek en therapeutische maatregelen naar aanleiding van de kursussen door Prof W.Janda. Course notes, 1984

[8] Butler D. Mobilisation of the nervous system. Melbourne: Churchill Livingstone, 1991

[9] Barral J–P, Mercier P. Visceral manipulation. Seattle: Eastland Press, 1988

[10] Upledger J. Your inner physician and you, 1st edn. Berkely, California: North Atlantic Books, 1991

[11] Basmajian J, Nyberg R. Rational manual therapies, 1st edn. Baltimore: Williams and Wilkins, 1993

[12] Watson P, Kendall N. Assessing psychosocial yellow flags. In: Gifford L, ed. Topical Issues in Pain 2. Biopsychosocial assessment and management. Relationships and pain. Falmouth: CNS Press, 2000: 111–129

[13] Oliver M. Theories of disability in health practice and research. British Medical Journal 1998; 317:1446–1449

[14] McColl M, Bickenbach J. Introduction. In: McColl M, Bickenbach J, eds. Introduction to disability. London: WB Saunders, 1998: 3–10

[15] Waddell G. The back pain revolution. Edinburgh: Churchill Livingstone, 1998

[16] Walker J, Holloway I, Sofaer B. In the system: the lived experience of chronic back pain from the perspectives of those seeking help from pain clinics. Pain 1999; 80:621–628

[17] Bigos S, Batti'e M, Spengler D, Fisher L, Fordyce W, Hansson T, et al. A longitudinal prospective study of industrial back injury. Clinical Orthopaedics 1992; 279:21–34

[18] Fordyce W. Back pain in the workplace. Management of disability in nonspecific conditions. Seattle: IASP Press, 1995

[19] Waddell G, Newton M, Henderson I, Sommerville D, Main C. A fear–avoidance beliefs questionnaire (FABQ) and the role of fear–avoidance in chronic low back pain and disability. Pain 1993; 52:157–168

[20] Harding V, Williams ACdC. Extending physiotherapy skills using a psychological approach: cognitive–behavioural management of chronic pain. Physiotherapy 1995; 81:11681–11688

[21] Morley S, Eccleston C, Williams ACdC. Systematic review and meta-analysis of randomized controlled trials of cognitive behaviour therapy and behaviour therapy for chronic pain in adults, excluding headache. Pain 1999; 80:1,21–13

[22] Wolff M, Hoskins Michel T, Krebs D. Chronic pain – assessment of orthopedic physical therapist's knowledge and attitudes. Phys Ther 1991; 71:207–214

[23] Harstall C, Ospina M. How prevalent is chronic pain? Pain – Clinical Updates 2003; XI 2

[24] Gifford L. Pain, the tissues and the nervous system: A conceptual model. Physiotherapy 1998; 84:127–136

[25] Greening J, Lynn B, Leary R. Sensory and autonomic function in the hands of patients with non-specific arm pain (NSAP) and asymptomatic office workers. Pain 2003; 104:1,2275–2282.

[26] Greening J, Lynn B. Minor peripheral nerve injuries: an underestimated source of pain? Man Ther 1998; 3:4187–4194

[27] Gifford L. The clinical biology of aches and pains. Falmouth: Neuro Orthopaedic Institute UK, 1996

[28] Boden S, Davis D, Dina T, et al. Abnormal magnetic resonance scans of the lumbar spine in asymptomatic subjects: a prospective investigation. J Bone Joint Surg (Am) 1990; 78(A):114–124

Nociceptive pain

Let us then suppose the Mind to be, as we say, white Paper void of all Characters without any Ideas: How comes it to be furnished?

JOHN LOCKE

INTRODUCTION

Pain arising from joints and soft tissues is a common reason for a visit to the manual therapist. This is the type of pain that therapists are most comfortable with, because it behaves and responds in the way predicted by the mechanical models. When force is applied to affected tissues the pain gets worse, while anything that offloads them relieves the pain.

Certain tissue events cause pain because they activate afferents specialized in the detection of *somatic* problems or problems in the body (see Glossary). These so-called *nociceptive nerves* are activated by extreme stimuli such as strong pressure or stretch, but also tissue damage and inflammation. Most musculoskeletal therapies aim to take away the factors that activate the nociceptive nerves in order to alleviate pain.

Most of this book deals with sources of pain outside the musculo-skeletal system. However, in order to determine whether treatment of the tissues is sufficient or whether other factors need to be addressed, the characteristics of nociceptive pain must be understood. Moreover, sometimes pain manifests in the somatic tissues but does not originate there. Only a clear understanding of the generation and characteristics of nociceptive pain enables the clinician to distinguish between different types of pain. This is important, because the wrong interpretation leads to the wrong treatment.

The word nociception is derived from the Latin word *nocere*, to damage. It is sensation as a result of the activation of specialized receptors at the end of nociceptive nerves, the so-called *nociceptors*. Nociceptive pain is pain as a result of the activation of nociceptors. It could be called *normal pain*, pain in the classic sense of the word, in absence of any psychological influence and without damage of the nervous system.

However, although the body has this specialized damage detection system, pain is not necessarily the consequence of nociception, as

Box 2.1 Illustration of pain without nociception

The following story was reported in the medical literature.[1] A builder falls and a 15 cm nail is driven through his foot. The pain is excruciating. His colleagues try to remove it from his foot, but the man is in too much agony. In the end they decide to take him to the local emergency department with the nail in situ. The extreme pain prevents emergency doctors from removing it, so they put the victim under sedation. When they finally remove nail and boot, they are astounded. The nail is located in the space between the first and second toe, not causing any damage at all.

illustrated in Box 2.1. Pain can exist in absence of nociception, and nociception does not inevitably lead to pain.

The definition of pain used by the International Association for the Study of Pain is: 'An unpleasant sensory and emotional experience associated with actual or potential tissue damage, or described in terms of such damage.' This definition includes two types of tissue-based pain, actual and potential. The first type is pain as a result of tissue damage, the second is the result of a stimulus that has the potential to *become* damaging if sustained or increased. Each of these involves particular types of receptors and afferents and each has particular characteristics that can be recognized in the clinical setting.

This chapter describes how tissue damage and inflammation can generate pain through the stimulation of certain afferents. In order to clarify some paradoxical characteristics of the sensory nerves, the evolution of the nervous system is introduced. This evolutionary theme recurs in several successive chapters.

An explanation of how inflammation does not just stimulate nociceptive nerves but is in fact regulated by it, is included. The regulation of tissue healing is introduced, but is expanded on in Chapter 5. Finally, characteristics of nociceptive pain are discussed in order to empower the clinician to distinguish this type of pain from others and select the appropriate treatment.

DETECTION OF TISSUE EVENTS

The following section is based on references.[2-4]

Physiologically, anything that happens to the body's tissues can lead to awareness only if it triggers a response in the nervous system. This response starts in the peripheral terminals of sensory nerves, where stimuli lead to the generation of electrical signals. Stimuli important for the musculoskeletal therapies are mechanical in nature, for example stretch, pressure and vibration. Examples of non-mechanical stimuli are cooling or warming of the tissues, tissue injury and the release of chemicals.

Generally speaking, the physiological role of the peripheral sensory nerve is to generate signals in response to events in the tissues and conduct these signals to the central nervous system. In the spinal cord, enormous amounts of sensory input are received, processed and passed on to the brain.

Although each type of stimulus affects the afferents in a unique way, the underlying principles are the same. A neurone will generate a signal only when the electrical voltage across its membrane is lowered to a certain level, as detailed in Box 2.2. Therefore, all tissue events must somehow lead to the reduction of this electrical voltage, even though they are not electrical in nature themselves. This transformation of mechanical, thermal and chemical stimuli into electrical signals is called *transduction*.

Transduction takes place in receptors at the peripheral end of sensory nerves. There are different types of receptor, each specialized to

When a nerve is at rest, the outside of its membrane has a more positive electrical charge than the inside. This *resting potential* is the result of the distribution of ions with positive and negative charges, namely sodium, potassium and chloride. The membrane of the nerve contains gates for each type of ion called *ion channels*, which are closed in the resting state.

Each ion channel can be opened by a specific influence (Fig. 2.1). Ligand-gated channels open when a specific chemical from outside the nerve called a *ligand* binds with it. A ligand works like a key in a lock. Other channels, which are important for the response to stretch and compression, are pulled open by mechanical forces. A third category is the voltage-gated channel, which opens when the electrical potential across the nerve's membrane changes beyond a certain threshold level.

When ion channels open in response to a chemical, mechanical or electrical influence, ions flow through them and change the electrical charge of the nerve locally. As soon as this charge reaches the threshold for local voltage gated ion channels, they open as well, increasing the ion flow considerably. This creates an *action potential*, a reversal of the electrical charge, which is the nerve's response to the stimulus (Fig. 2.2).

The generation of an action potential follows an all-or-nothing principle: if the threshold level is not reached the nerve will not respond, but when threshold is reached it will. There is no in-between state, so a stronger stimulation does not result in a greater depolarization. However, the nerve is able to respond to increasing levels of stimulation by increasing the frequency at which it generates action potentials.

When an action potential is generated somewhere along the nerve, the neighbouring voltage-gated ion channels respond to the change in electrical charge. This leads to a repetition of the same process and the generation of another action potential. This process is repeated along the whole nerve and forms the basis for its conduction of signals.

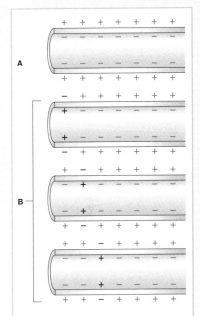

Fig. 2.2 The generation and propagation of an action potential. At rest, the inside of a nerve is more negatively charged than its surroundings. The opening of ion channels reverses the charge (action potential). Subsequent opening of adjacent ion channels propagates the action potential.

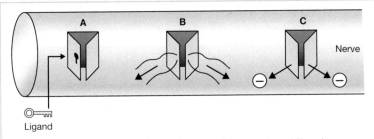

Fig. 2.1. Ion channels. Channels may be opened by an external ligand **A**, a mechanical force **B**, or an electrical charge **C**.

respond to a particular type of stimulus. *Mechanoreceptors* contain ion channels that can be pulled open when a certain mechanical force is applied to them. Each *chemoreceptor* responds when a specific chemical binds to it. *Thermal receptors* are activated by changes in temperature. Finally, the so-called *nociceptors* respond to injury, inflammation and stimuli that have the potential to damage. Although some nociceptors are specialized for a certain type of stimulus, many are *polymodal* or responsive to several kinds of stimuli, specifically thermal, chemical and mechanical.

The general classification of A alpha–delta, B and C is based on the measurement of conduction speed. Sensory researchers however, prefer to use classes I to IV based on diameter and receptor innervation because they are easier to verify than conduction speed. Differences between nociceptive fibres are detailed in Table 2.1.

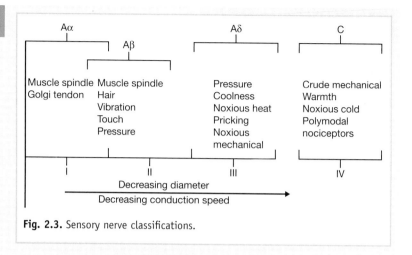

Fig. 2.3. Sensory nerve classifications.

SENSORY NERVE FIBRES

Each type of receptor is *expressed* or produced by a specific type of afferent. With the exception of moderate cooling and warming, sensations that do not threaten tissue integrity are mediated by thick, fast-conducting myelinated fibres. On the other hand, all nociceptors are part of much thinner and therefore much slower fibres. The thin fibres of group A delta have a myelin sheath, whereas C fibres are unmyelinated. Box 2.3 gives an overview of sensory nerve classifications.* (Fig. 2.3)

There are a few important functional differences between nociceptors and other receptors. First, because nociceptors have a much higher stimulation threshold they usually do not respond unless they are subjected to an intense stimulus. Second, as a group they are much less stimulus specific than non-noxious receptors, because many nociceptors are polymodal or sensitive to mechanical, thermal and chemical stimuli. Finally, many non-noxious receptors adapt to ongoing stimulation. For example, paciniform mechanoreceptors demonstrate a structural adjustment to constant pressure as well as an accommodation of the afferent itself.[4] On the other hand, nociceptors keep firing or may even become more sensitive.

These response qualities are important for the organism as a whole. Nociceptive neurones form part of a system that raises the alert when there is a current or impending physical problem. They do not need to become active under normal circumstances. When they do, the priority is to react rather than to analyse the exact nature of the stimulus, so specificity is not important. Finally, adaptation is the nervous system's way of cancelling information that does not require attention such as the feel of clothes or a ticking clock, but noxious stimulation is important at all times.

Thermal nociceptors are innervated by A delta and C fibres and signal extreme heat and cold. They create a sensation of burning or

*This classification does not apply to visceral sensation, which is mostly mediated by C fibres. Visceral and musculoskeletal sensations are quite different from each other. Viscera are often insensitive to sensations that cause pain in somatic tissues. For example, the bowel can be cut without the slightest discomfort, but distension can be extremely painful.

Table 2.1 Comparison of the characteristics of A delta and C fibres. Characteristics referred to by the letter a are physiological, while b describes the consequences for the nature of the pain

Characteristic	A delta	C
1a. Conduction speed	Fast (4–36m/s)	Slow (0.4–2m/s)
1b. Pain onset	First/fast pain	Second/slow pain
2a. Accommodation (adaptation)	Fast	Slow
2b. Pain duration	Brief	Long
3a. Receptive field	Small	Large
3b. Localization	Precise	Diffuse
4. Sensory quality	Sharp, pricking	Aching, dull, burning
5. CNS response	Reflex, analysis	Emotional, suffering

freezing. A delta fibres innervate mechanical nociceptors, while polymodal nociceptors are innervated by C fibres. Polymodal receptors can respond to thermal, mechanical and chemical stimuli. They form the largest group of nociceptors.

The differences between A delta and C fibres give rise to what is sometimes referred to as 'the duality of pain'. When a painful stimulus activates both types of nerve (the adventurous reader may try hammering a small nail into the non-dominant hand to observe this), each conveys a particular aspect of the stimulus. Table 2.1 gives an overview of the differences.

The information conveyed by A delta fibres can be described as more analytical than C fibre mediated information. Because it is brief, well localized and fast, it allows quick and accurate analysis of the source of nociception. At the beginning of the 20th century, the English neurologist Henry Head proposed the term 'epicritic sensibility' to describe this type of nociception, a term that is still in use.[5,6] In contrast, pain mediated by C fibres is much less specific, as is the response it creates. Someone who hits his thumb with a hammer will first respond in a reflex action and next realize exactly that the thumb was hit. It hurts, but the initial A delta pain is manageable – until the slow C fibre pain comes in, making the victim double over and wanting to cry.[2] Head introduced the term 'protopathic sensibility' for this more diffuse type of sensation.

Price describes a number of historical experiments that have confirmed the relative contributions of A delta and C fibres to the perception of pain.[7] Selective stimulation of A delta fibres enables only the perception of sharp, brief, well-localized sensations, while a selective blockade of all myelinated fibres preserves only deep, diffuse pains with a burning quality. The latter can be observed in everyday life (Box 2.4).

Box 2.4 An experiment to demonstrate pain qualities associated with the stimulation of different types of nociceptive fibre

Price suggests a simple experiment, involving the exertion of sustained pressure on the ulnar nerve, which can be done by lying supine with the arms by one's sides.[8] An alternative is the application of a blood pressure cuff inflated to above systolic pressure for around 30 minutes.[9] Because large diameter fibres are more dependent on the blood supply than unmyelinated fibres, A beta fibres are knocked out first, followed by A delta fibres, finally leaving only C fibres functioning. When the sensitivity to light touch first disappears, i.e. when A beta fibres stop functioning, a quick sharp pinch evokes a change in pain sensation. Once the skin becomes very numb because all myelinated fibres have stopped working, the same pinch causes a delayed pain that outlasts the pinch, feels dull and has a somewhat burning quality.

Early sensory research concentrated on the identification of specific receptors and afferents for each type of sensation.[9] It is now clear that this elusive one-on-one relationship does not exist. Any stimulus activates a variety of receptor types, each of which registers a particular aspect of the stimulus. In other words, the stimulus is deconstructed into elements that our nervous system recognizes. Once all signals arrive in the brain, they are re-integrated to create a sensation. This is also where they are given meaning, which is one of the factors that determines the difference between for example a painful stretch applied by a trusted clinician and a similar pain when lifting a heavy object (see Box 2.5). The first is perceived as a pain that will ultimately be beneficial, whereas the latter sets off alarm bells.

AN EVOLUTIONARY MODEL OF THE NERVOUS SYSTEM

It may seem strange that very efficient myelinated fibres conduct gentle stimuli that don't pose any threat to us, while noxious stimulation activates slow and diffuse systems. A model that makes this apparent contradiction easier to understand is based on the theory that throughout the evolution of the species, more efficient systems developed in order to improve the chances of survival. This model also provides a useful way of remembering the functional characteristics of the three types of sensory afferent.

Thin, unmyelinated fibres can be thought of as primitive and *phylogenetically* old, i.e. old in terms of evolution. They have the most basic structure of all nerves and are slow conducting. The information that these C fibres yield is very non-specific because of their characteristics. The first characteristic concerns timing. C fibres have a delayed response that develops slowly and takes time to settle down again. The second factor is the polymodal nature of the receptors that does not allow an analysis of the exact nature of the stimulus. Finally, the large receptive field makes localization of the stimulus difficult. The response evoked by C-fibre stimulation comes from the phylogenetically older, emotional brain. It is an: 'I don't like this, whatever it is' response. It promotes a general change in behaviour rather than a stimulus-specific response.

The next step in sensory evolution is the development of A delta fibres. They are still thin, but a myelin sheath makes them more efficient. Specialized receptors enable an analysis of the exact nature of the noxious stimulus. A delta fibres are fast and have a small receptive field, making possible a reflex that is stimulus-specific. They give details about the timing of a noxious stimulus, because their response is quick and does not last beyond stimulation. A delta fibres are linked with the analytical parts of the brain.

Both A delta and C fibres have a high stimulation threshold, so that only unpleasant stimuli get through to the central nervous system. They are part of an alarm system, which is to a large extent purely reactive: it is activated only when stimuli become excessive. In order to develop further, species need an even more refined sensory system

---

Box 2.5 Painful musculoskeletal therapies

Manual treatments can be somewhat unpleasant, but there are several aspects that enable an experienced clinician to control the nociceptive stimulation. First, there tends to be a simultaneous A beta stimulation when a technique is applied well, for example by the mechanical stimulation of placing one's hands on the patient's body. As demonstrated in the experiment of Box 2.3, A beta fibres moderate the pain perception. Second, most painful therapeutic techniques tend to stimulate A delta, but not C fibres. For instance, the pain caused by manually pressing an active trigger point is sharp and intense, but it eases in less than 90 seconds. These qualities suggest A delta fibre stimulation. C fibres produce pain of a different quality and a longer duration. They also produce a more non-specific and emotional reaction, which may be counterproductive in a musculoskeletal clinic. Finally, the clinician provides meaning to the brain by explaining what causes the pain, by reassuring the patient that it will be temporary and by generally instilling confidence. The way the brain and therefore the person interprets a painful sensation has a very powerful effect on its impact, a principle that will be revisited several times in this book. Meaning forms part of any treatment and should never be ignored.

in the form of fast myelinated A beta fibres. With their highly specialized receptors, they perceive subtle changes such as light touch. Species with C and A delta fibres as the only sensory fibres can react to unpleasant stimuli, but cannot be aware of much else. With the development of low threshold A beta fibres, pain can be anticipated and avoided, because the increase of a stimulus is felt before it reaches noxious levels.

In the evolutionary model, newer and more specific systems do not replace the older ones. Instead they are superimposed, exerting a moderating influence on previously developed systems. An example is the plantar withdrawal reflex, assessed in the Babinski test. The phylogenetically primitive structures responsible for this reflex are present in everyone's spinal cord, but the influence of higher order centres suppresses their activation. However, when this controlling influence is taken away, for instance because of spinal cord damage or a stroke, the reflex returns.

Another example of superimposition is the moderating influence that new sensory systems have on older ones. When A delta fibres are knocked out in the experiment described in Box 2.4, the C fibre response is more intense and lasts longer. One could say that the old response has become more controlled because of the presence of the new system. The introduction of a third system in the form of A beta fibres enables even more control, as described in Melzack and Wall's Gate Theory of pain control (see Ch. 4). Put simply, noxious stimulation caused by walking into the edge of a desk can be eased by rubbing the skin, which provides A beta stimulation.

The disadvantage of evolutionary development is increasing vulnerability. Old cars may not be as fast and efficient as modern cars with electronic engine management systems, but pliers and screwdriver are often sufficient to repair them. Primitive life forms may not be very sophisticated, but they are extremely resilient. C fibres are simple in structure and therefore resistant to damage and easily regenerated. In comparison, thick myelinated fibres are vulnerable to mechanical influences. Their regeneration process is fraught with difficulty, as will become clear in the next chapter.

HOW DO TISSUE EVENTS ACTIVATE NOCICEPTORS?

Two types of process can lead to the generation of an action potential in a nociceptive neurone (Fig. 2.4). When a stimulus generates an action potential, the nerve is activated. Some would say that the nerve fires. However, other influences merely lower the membrane potential of the nerve. While this in itself may not be sufficient to generate an action potential, it will make the nerve more easily excitable when subjected to another stimulus. This is referred to as *sensitization*.

For example, if a person's forearm is being squeezed a considerable amount of pressure is required to make it hurt, because the mechanical and polymodal nociceptors have a high stimulation threshold. However, if that person has a fresh bruise on their forearm much less pressure is

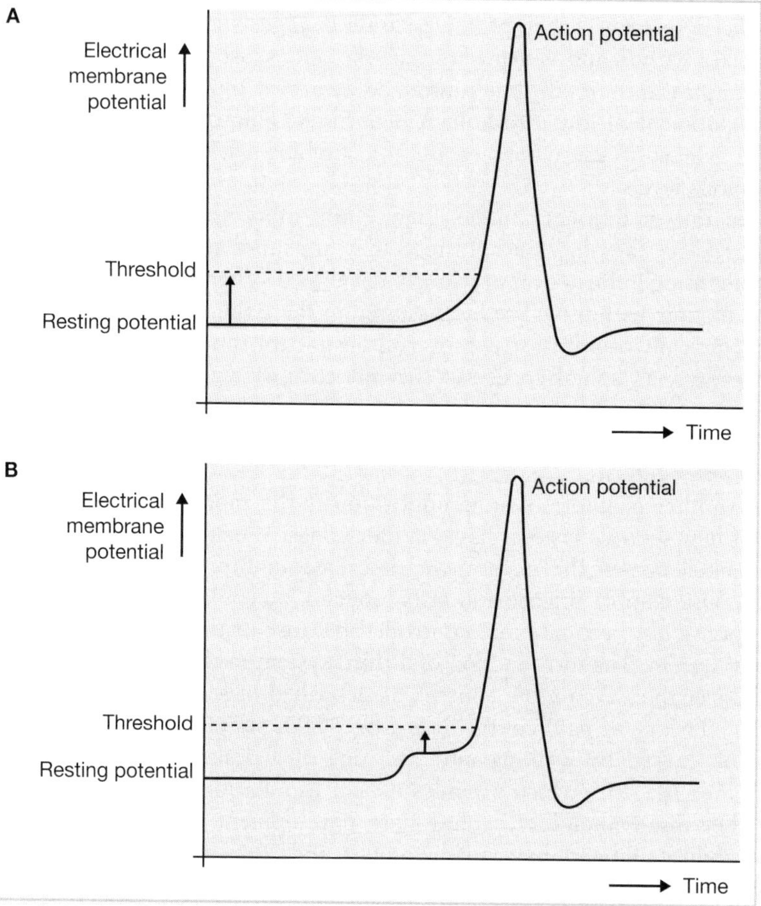

Fig. 2.4 Sensitization of a sensory nerve. A stimulus of certain strength is required to lower the membrane potential to threshold level and generate an action potential. Sensitization lowers the membrane potential, bringing it closer to threshold but not necessarily sufficiently to depolarize the nerve. However, the sensitized nerve now depolarizes in response to a much weaker stimulus.

required to cause the nociceptive fibres to respond, even if the bruise does not hurt spontaneously. The reason is that the nerve endings in the area of the bruise have been sensitized, i.e. their membrane potential has been lowered and brought closer to threshold level.

Even a moderate amount of pressure that is normally not sufficient to cause pain can be painful when it is applied to a bruise or otherwise sensitized area. When a normally innocuous stimulus is sufficient to cause pain, this is referred to as *allodynia*. Because there may be sensitivity to one type of stimulus but not another, it is important to be specific in one's notes by for instance writing 'cold allodynia' or 'allodynia to light touch'.*

Sensitized afferents also respond more strongly to stimuli that would be expected to be painful even under normal circumstances, by generating action potentials at a higher rate. This is called *hyperalgesia*, and when it is the result of sensitization in the periphery the term *primary hyperalgesia* is used.*

Stimulation and sensitization are the mechanisms responsible for the generation of pain and local tenderness when tissues are damaged

*Secondary hyperalgesia is the result of changes in the central nervous system rather than the periphery and will be discussed in Chapter 4.

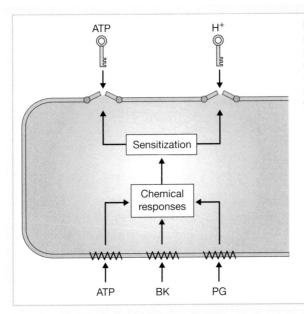

Fig. 2.5 Mechanisms of inflammatory pain. Inflammatory mediators such as hydrogen (H^+), adenosine triphosphate (ATP), bradykinin (BK) and prostaglandins (PG) bind with receptors on ion channels, which open and cause the membrane potential to change. They also bind with metabotropic receptors that change the internal response of the nerve and the sensitivity of the ion channels.

or inflamed (for an overview of the mechanisms involved, see for example[17]). Histamine is an example of a chemical that activates nociceptive neurones directly and causes pain in absence of other stimuli. Other chemicals such as prostaglandins, adenosine triphosphate (ATP) and bradykinin sensitize the nerve endings, making activation more likely. These processes are not fully understood, but can be summarized as follows (Fig. 2.5).

Activation of a nerve requires the flow of ions across its membrane, which happens when ion channels open. The ligand gated ion channels in nociceptive nerve endings open when certain chemicals (ligands) bind to their receptors, comparable to turning a key in a lock to open a door. Because in this case the receptor is part of the ion channel, this mechanism is referred to as 'direct gating'. Ligands for the ion channels in nociceptors include ATP, hydrogen ions and capsaicin, the 'hot' chemical in chilli peppers.

Sensitization is the result of the binding of, for example, prostaglandin E2, bradykinin, adrenaline and ATP to a different type of receptor. This so-called metabotropic receptor is not linked to an ion channel directly, but it can start a process inside the nerve that makes ion channels easier to activate.

Nociceptive neurones are commonly activated and sensitized by tissue damage and the subsequent inflammatory processes.

TISSUE DAMAGE AND INFLAMMATION

When tissues are damaged, a sequence of events is set in motion, ideally resulting in repair of the damaged structures. This sequence can be divided into three overlapping stages (Fig. 2.6). Inflammation

Fig. 2.6 Waxing and waning of inflammatory, proliferative and regenerative processes following injury (based on [17]).

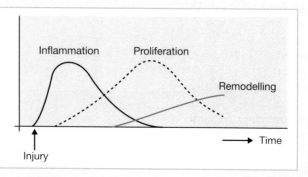

starts very soon after injury and reaches its peak within days. As the inflammatory process begins to reduce, proliferation of cells involved in cleaning up and repairing the area builds up. This phase peaks after a few weeks and gradually subsides as the final stage develops. During this remodelling stage the tissues are strengthened.

The clinical signs of inflammation were first described by the Roman Celcus in (fl AD c. 30) as rubor (redness), calor (warmth), tumor (swelling) and dolor (pain).[11] These signs can be observed in most patients with acute lesions and are explained by the sequence of events following injury.

When soft tissue cells are damaged, they disintegrate and release a number of chemicals. These chemicals, for example potassium ions, bind with receptors on nociceptive nerves and generate action potentials.[12] This is how tissue damage causes immediate pain.

Some of the released substances are enzymes, which in turn lead to the release of so-called *inflammatory mediators* such as histamine, bradykinin and several types of prostaglandin from local cells. As discussed in the previous section, these chemicals are potent generators of nociceptive pain.

If capillaries in the tissues are damaged, the supply of oxygen is disrupted. The immediate result is ischaemic pain (for the mechanism of ischaemic pain, please see reference [12]). In addition, lack of oxygen leads to further cell death and a subsequent increase in concentrations of inflammatory mediators. The blood vessels that are still intact respond to the inflammatory mediators with vasodilation, increasing the blood flow and causing the area to become red and warm.

As the vessels dilate, their endothelial cells separate. The combination of increased flow and greater permeability forces plasma proteins out of the capillaries and into the interstitial space. The result is an increase in colloid osmotic pressure, which draws more fluid into the interstitium and causes local swelling. All the signs classically associated with inflammation, i.e. redness, warmth, swelling and pain are now present.

The following section gives a brief overview of the remainder of the process of inflammation and healing. Platelets in the blood break and release thrombin, which mediates a reaction leading to the formation of a mesh of fibrin. This process is referred to as *walling off* the damaged area. The meshwork encapsulates the damaged cells and forms a clot. It reduces fluid flow to a minimum and prevents spread of toxic material and bacteria. At the same time, bacterial and cellular chemicals attract a series of white blood cells to the area. Together with the macrophages they clear away debris from damaged cells.

It takes 3–5 days for the inflammation to reach its peak. As the inflammatory response declines, repair of the damaged tissues starts in the proliferation phase (Box 2.6).

During the proliferation phase, capillaries grow towards the damaged area and start supplying oxygen, proteins and fluids, essential for the formation of new tissues. New lymphatic vessels grow, forming a drainage system for metabolites and waste products. At the same time, fibroblasts are drawn to the area. They form collagen and repair the connective tissues. The result is the formation of highly vascularized granulation tissue or scar tissue.

Fibroblasts are transformed into myofibroblasts, which have the capacity to contract. In doing so, they draw the edges of the wound together. Capillaries gradually reduce in number as the new tissue matures. Finally, the new tissue is strengthened in a process called remodelling. New collagen fibres are laid down in the direction of the tension the repairing area is subjected to, giving functional tensile strength to the newly formed tissue. Even when the healing process appears to be complete, remodelling may continue for several months. At this stage, exercises and manual interventions that impose a mechanical force on the tissue in a functional direction are thought to help to restore its strength. The force imposed on the tissue has to be appropriate for the strength of the new tissue.

NEURAL REGULATION OF INFLAMMATION

Nociceptive nerves produce chemicals called *neuropeptides* in their cell bodies. These neuropeptides are transported to the nerve's peripheral terminal, where they are stored. When the nerve receives a stimulus that is strong enough for it to depolarize, for instance when an injury is sustained, it releases the neuropeptides into the tissues it innervates.

The most described neuropeptides are *Substance P* (SP) and *Calcitonin Gene Related Peptide* (CGRP). They cause a local vasodilation, both by acting on the capillaries and by causing mast cells to release histamine. Histamine also sensitizes nerve endings in the area. These reactions were originally described by Lewis as the *Triple Response* (Thomas Lewis 1881–1945[11]) (Box 2.7).

The effects of SP and CGRP are potent enough to cause and maintain an inflammatory response in absence of any tissue damage. When this happens, it is referred to as a *neurogenic inflammation*,[8] which forms the basis of the hypothesis that rheumatoid arthritis may be mediated by the nervous system.[14]

Box 2.6

The proliferation phase does not just succeed inflammation, but is brought forth by it. As a result, an incomplete or slow inflammatory process leads to difficulties in tissue healing. The use of non-steroidal anti-inflammatory drugs (NSAIDs) in the first few days following an injury is therefore controversial. These drugs inhibit the formation of prostaglandins, thereby reducing the inflammatory response and potentially inhibiting tissue healing. In the first few days following an injury, it may be better to use paracetamol, which does not have an anti-inflammatory action. The patient can turn to NSAIDs if the inflammation persists.

Fig. 2.7 The axon reflex. Stimulation of a C fibre branch leads to depolarization of other branches and the release of neuropeptides in the surrounding area.

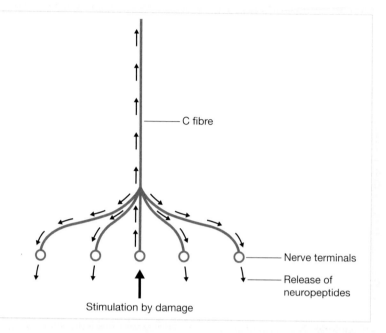

C fibre

Nerve terminals

Release of neuropeptides

Stimulation by damage

Box 2.7

Lewis' triple response can be observed when the skin is scratched or after a bee or wasp sting.[2,13] Mechanical deformation of the skin causes mast cells to release histamine, which makes the capillaries dilate. As a result, the scratch turns red.

Vasodilation makes the capillaries more permeable for proteins, which are pushed out of the vessels and into the surrounding space. The resulting change in colloid osmotic pressure draws fluids into the tissues, making the scratch swell and turn white.

High threshold afferents (nociceptive nerves) release neuropeptides and the area surrounding the scratch becomes red and sore.

The practical application of the triple response is the investigation of sensitization of the peripheral nociceptive nerves. If the sharp end of a reflex hammer is dragged over the skin, for instance along the spine, areas innervated by sensitized afferents are likely to show a heightened response. This provides useful diagnostic information about the peripheral nerve or spinal level involved.

The effects of neuropeptides are not just observed in the area that is affected directly, but also in the adjacent skin region (stage 3 of the triple response). This observation cannot be explained by the diffusion of vasodilatory chemicals released by the nerve endings. Instead, it is the result of the *axon reflex* (Fig. 2.7).[13] When a branch of a C fibre is stimulated, the resulting action potentials are transmitted to the central nervous system. Where they reach other branches, action potentials are also generated in those branches and sent to their terminals, being conducted as it were the 'wrong way' or *antidromically*. Once these antidromic action potentials reach the peripheral terminals, neuropeptides are released from these surrounding branches as well.

CHARACTERISTICS OF NOCICEPTIVE PAIN ORIGINATING IN THE MUSCULOSKELETAL TISSUES

As discussed in this chapter, some tissue events can generate action potentials in nociceptive neurones and lead to the perception of pain. Normally, these neurones have a high threshold and respond only to strong stimuli. However, damage and inflammation are associated with the release of chemicals that sensitize the nerve endings and make them more responsive. When the strong stimulus is withdrawn or the inflammatory mediators disappear, the afferents stop firing. These observations dictate the characteristics of clinical tissue based pain.

Description by the patient

- Nociceptive pain is consistent in its behaviour. It limits itself to one region and responds predictably.
- There are some postures or activities that consistently ease the pain, while others always make it worse.
- Rest helps to ease the pain.
- Inconsistencies in aggravating and easing factors suggest the involvement of other pain mechanisms. Severe and/or progressive pain without any easing factors is classed as a 'Red Flag' and requires investigation.[15]

Examination findings

- Pain resulting purely from the stimulation of high threshold afferents should respond to the mechanical force it is subjected to in a consistent way.
- Tests that mechanically offload the affected tissue can be expected to reduce the pain, while increased stretch or pressure should do the opposite. Tests of distant structures do not influence the pain. This is the basis of Cyriax' selective tissue tensioning and Edwards' combined movements, for example.
- Finally, there is well-localized hyperalgesia and allodynia on palpation but beware, soreness does not always mean that the palpated structure is the source of the pain!

Time course

- Pain resulting purely from mechanical forces should disappear when those forces are removed.
- Inflammation can be expected to resolve within weeks, unless it is part of a systemic condition such as rheumatoid arthritis.
- Pain that does not follow the expected time course may either be caused or maintained by other factors.

Response to medication

Non-steroidal anti-inflammatory drugs (NSAIDs) such as aspirin, Voltarol or Brufen reduce the release of prostaglandins, which are potent inflammatory mediators. If these drugs are taken after the peak of the suspected inflammatory phase and they fail to produce any pain relief, other pain mechanisms must be considered.

Response to physical treatment

Manual therapy and the prescription of appropriate exercise can be expected to have a beneficial effect on the mechanical status of the tissues, for example by improving their mobility or reducing the load they need to bear.

Box 2.8

Andrew, a car mechanic who owned his own garage, was admitted to hospital after he fractured his femur in a fall. Despite weeks with the appropriate treatment, his fracture failed to heal. Andrew was getting increasingly worried, because he was self-employed and there was no one to stand in for him. He could not afford to be in hospital and lose his customers, but he had no choice. He felt trapped.

One of the nurses looking after Andrew had a theory. Perhaps his emotional stress was preventing him from getting better. Instead of directing his energy inwards to his own body, he was directing it outwards, to a cause about which he could do nothing. It was a vicious cycle.

The nurse involved a social worker who contacted an employment agency. An unemployed mechanic agreed to run the garage until Andrew was well again. Andrew began to relax and resigned himself to his recovery period. A few weeks later, an X-ray of his femur demonstrated early signs of healing. Eventually, he recovered completely and returned to work.

Box 2.9. Brain teaser: does sustained mechanical strain cause pain?

Many therapists use a simple experiment to demonstrate to their patients that sustained mechanical force can cause pain if it is sustained for long enough. This experiment, suggested by Robin McKenzie, involves passively forcing a finger into hyperextension, initially without causing pain. When the same pressure is maintained for a few minutes, the finger begins to hurt. The therapists who use this experiment, usually explain that abnormal strains eventually lead to pain, even if they are not damaging.

The reader is invited to try the following experiment and compare the results with the previous one. Clench one fist as tightly as possible. After a short while, the hand becomes uncomfortable. Continue to clench the fist tightly. What happens after another minute or so? Do the observations confirm the conclusion from McKenzie's experiment, or do they require an alternative?

Fig. 2.8 Central regulation of circulation in musculoskeletal tissues. The sympathetic nervous system (SNS) secretes noradrenaline from its fibres, regulating circulation locally. It also stimulates the adrenal cortex to release adrenaline into the blood stream, which affects circulation more generally. The adrenal cortex also releases cortisol, which affects the availability of amino acids necessary for tissue regeneration.[4]

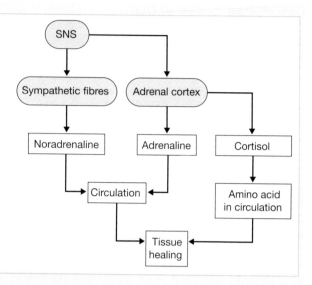

Some electrotherapy modalities are thought to aid the resolution of inflammation [17].

If the response to these interventions is absent or unpredictable, the therapist needs to revisit the original diagnosis or hypothesis.

Regulatory influences

Tissue damage and inflammation are a common cause of pain. From the description of the processes involved in the resolution of inflammation and the repair of tissue damage, it would seem that they are purely local and self-regulatory. Apart from the neuropeptides that fuel and speed up the inflammatory response, the role of the nervous system appears to be limited to that of the passive observer. However, in reality these local processes are influenced centrally. Because this central regulation is normally extremely efficient, it is easy to overlook its importance for the effective resolution of tissue pathology (see for example Box 2.8).

Essential constituents in the healing process are oxygen and proteins, both of which are supplied by the circulation. Circulation is regulated by local processes, but also by the sympathetic and adrenal system via the release of noradrenaline and adrenaline. These so-called *catecholamines* affect vasodilation and vasoconstriction. If the sympathetic nervous system is persistently active, for instance as a result of ongoing emotional stress, the capillaries may be prevented from responding to local demand. In addition, stress stimulates the release of the hormone cortisol, which leads to a reduction in the availability of proteins required for tissue repair.

The exact role of the sympathetic nervous system and related endocrine systems are the subject of Chapter 5, but their relevance for inflammation and healing is summarized in Figure 2.7.

References

[1] Fisher J, Hassan D, O'Connor N. Minerva. BMJ 1995; 310:70

[2] van Cranenburgh B. Pijn – vanuit een neurowetenschappelijk perspectief (Pain from a neuroscientific perspective). Maarssen: Elsevier Gezondheidszorg, 2000

[3] Kandel E. Principles of neural science, 4th edn. New York: McGraw-Hill, 2000

[4] Guyton A, Hall J. Textbook of medical physiology. Philadelphia: WB Saunders, 2000

[5] Head H, Holmes G. Studies in neurology. London: Frowde, Stodder and Houghton, 1920

[6] Gardner E, Martin J, Jessell T. The bodily senses. In: Kandel E, Schwartz J, Jessell T, eds. Principles of neural science. New York: McGraw-Hill, 2000: 430–450

[7] Price D. Psychological mechanisms of pain and analgesia. Seattle: IASP Press, 1999

[8] Basbaum A, Jessell T. The perception of pain. In: Kandel E, Schwartz J, Jessell T, eds. Principles of neural science. New York: McGraw-Hill, 2000: 472-491

[9] Sinclair D. Mechanisms of cutaneous sensation, 2nd edn. Oxford: Oxford University Press, 1981

[10] Kidd B, Urban L. Mechanisms of inflammatory pain. British Journal of Anaesthesia 2001; 87(1):311

[11] Porter R. The greatest benefit to mankind. A medical history of humanity from antiquity to the present. New York: HarperCollins, 1997

[12] Sutherland S, Cook S, McCleskey E. Chemical mediators of pain due to tissue damage and ischemia. Prog Brain Res 2000; 129:21–38

[13] de Morree J. Dynamiek van het menselijk bindweefsel. Functie, beschadiging en herstel. Utrecht: Bohn, Scheltema and Holkema, 1989

[14] Levine J, Collier D, Basbaum A, Moskowitz M, Helms C. Hypothesis: the nervous system may contribute to the pathophysiology of rheumatoid arthritis. J Rheumatol 1985; 12(3):406–409

[15] Clinical Standards Advisory Group. CSAG Report on low back pain. 1994: 1–89

[16] Maitland G. Vertebral Manipulation 5th edn. London, Butterworths, 1986

[17] Watson T. Soft tissue wound healing review. www.electrotherapy.org/modalities.htm.10-4-05

CONCLUSION

Although a patient may suggest that a muscle hurts, it can be argued that it is the brain that hurts. The injured muscle merely generates impulses in nociceptive nerves, but the brain may or may not interpret these impulses as pain. The characteristics of the pain enable the clinician to answer the following questions.

Is the pain consistently nociceptive in its presentation? This can be done by following Maitland's advice to persistently 'make features fit', i.e. making sure that the hypothesis of the cause of the pain explains all its subjective and objective characteristics.[17] If there are features that fall outside the tissue model, then the hypothesis needs to be expanded. For instance, there may be minor nerve damage or altered pain perception in the central nervous system. The rest of this book is devoted to the task of finding an explanatory model that fits the patient's signs and symptoms.

If the answer to the first question is yes, i.e. the nociceptive pain model explains the patient's signs and symptoms consistently, the following question has to be answered: do non-local factors need to be included in order to facilitate the recovery process? As discussed in the previous section, even when pain is the result of a localized soft tissue lesion the healing process relies on a number of central factors. Some of the successes of non-specific treatment techniques such as relaxation or Chi Kung may be based on their influence on autonomic and endocrine function.

For those readers who are certain that they understand the way mechanical forces generate pain, a 'brain teaser' is given in Box 2.8.

Peripheral neurogenic pain

Just because you feel it, doesn't mean it's there.

RADIOHEAD, *HAIL TO THE THIEF*

INTRODUCTION

The previous chapter described how tissue pathology is detected by peripheral nociceptive neurones, which in turn transmit information to the central nervous system. Ultimately, this information reaches the brain, where conscious awareness of the pathology arises. Under normal circumstances, the sensation arising in the brain can be expected to be congruent with the events in the tissues. In other words, what the person feels will mirror what is happening in their body. The nervous system merely passes on information, analogous to a telephone cable passing on the spoken word. This means that low intensity stimuli affect A beta fibres and generate normal non-painful sensation. For example, touch is perceived as touch and stretch as stretch. The intensity of the felt sensation corresponds with the intensity of the stimulus. Once the stimulus intensity reaches threatening levels, a dedicated nociceptive system is activated.

A requirement for the congruency between somatic pathology and pain is that the peripheral nerves function in a consistent way. The telephone line is expected to pass on each variation in pitch and volume without distortion, otherwise the person on the other end will find it difficult to make sense of what is being said. Similarly, if disturbances in nerve function interfere with the transmission of information from the tissues to the brain, the brain will have difficulties interpreting what is happening somatically.

Interestingly, this is where the telecommunications analogy ends. Whereas it is usually easy for someone to decide that there is a bad telephone connection, the brain is not very good at working out the difference between somatic pathology and a disturbance in nerve function. As a result, signals from nociceptive neurones are usually interpreted as a sign of tissue pathology, even when they are the result of problems in the peripheral nerve (the connection or line) (Fig. 3.1).

When pathology affects the afferents innervating the musculoskeletal tissues rather than those tissues themselves, one or several of the following phenomena can occur.

Fig. 3.1 The brain all information coming through nociceptive nerves as signs of tissue pathology.

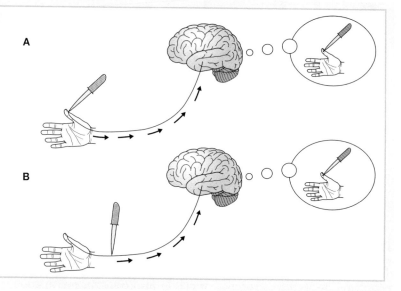

- If the nerve is severely damaged, signals from the periphery are interrupted. Although numbness and a loss of pain sensation seems the obvious and inevitable result of nerve damage, other more mysterious symptoms may also arise.
- Malfunctioning or damaged nerves often distort information from the periphery, misinforming the brain about what is going on in the body.
- Malfunctioning or damaged nerves may generate signals of their own accord, in absence of stimulation in the periphery. As explained above, the brain has little option but to interpret these signals as coming from the periphery.

This chapter focuses on *peripheral neurogenic/neuropathic pain*, or pain arising from problems in peripheral nerves. Although this type of pain *manifests* in the tissues and can therefore easily be mistaken as being caused by the tissues, it is in fact very different in aetiology. Because neurogenic pain mechanisms are very different from those involved in tissue damage and inflammation, the treatments are different as well. Consequently, it is essential for clinicians to be able to differentiate between somatic and neurogenic problems, if they want to target the source of the symptoms more accurately. The difference between neurogenic and neuropathic pain, although not clinically relevant, is discussed below under Peripheral neurogenic and neuropathic pain.

RECOVERY AFTER FRANK NERVE DAMAGE

The English neurologist Henry Head studied nerve damage by carefully observing his patients around the beginning of the 20th century. However, 'It soon became obvious that many observed facts would remain inexplicable without experimentation carried out more carefully and for a longer period than was possible with a patient, however willing...It is also unwise to demand any but the simplest introspection from patients, to whatever class they may belong.'[2]

Head decided to study the effects of peripheral sensory nerve damage in a classic experiment, which can be repeated by the interested reader under medical supervision. He had his own lateral antebrachial cutaneous nerve cut at the elbow and meticulously recorded signs and symptoms over a long period following this transection. The results made it clear that neural recovery is more complicated than that of the soft tissues. If neural recovery were similar, it could be expected to progress from numbness via returning sensation to normal sensation. Instead, nerve recovery is associated with seemingly contradictory changes, summed up in Box 3.2.

The non-linear process of neural healing can be explained by the recovery rates of different types of afferents (Fig. 3.3). It makes it clear that each type of nerve contributes to normal sensation. The following discussion is simplified by describing the recovery of nerve types C and A beta underlying the observations from Box 3.2.

DEVELOPMENT OF A HYPERPATHIC BORDER REGION
(Fig. 3.3.A)

There is a central zone of complete loss of sensation, as can be expected after denervation. However, the innervation fields of unmyelinated neurones from adjacent nerves overlap slightly. The perimeter of the denervated cutaneous region is therefore still innervated by C fibres from neighbouring, undamaged nerves. The result is a completely denervated centre and a narrow ring with nothing but nociceptive innervation.

Inward spread of hyperpathia (Fig. 3.3.B)

Macrophages and other cells in the area of damage release nerve growth factor (NGF).[4] This so-called *neurotrophic factor* causes the C fibres from intact neighbouring nerves to grow into the denervated area, a process called *collateral sprouting*. As a result, the area with innervation from nociceptive but not A beta fibres spreads inwards.

Normalization of sensation in the border region
(Fig. 3.3.C)

NGF causes collateral sprouting of neighbouring myelinated fibres as well. This takes place at a slower rate, because the structure and recovery process of these fibres are more complex. As they reach the area of altered sensation, they begin to normalize the balance of thin and thick fibres. This balance is required for normal sensation. The circumference of the hyperpathic area shrinks as a result of the normalizing distribution of afferents.

Box 3.1 The functional makeup of peripheral nerves

The somatic tissues are innervated by peripheral nerves, which originate in the spinal cord. These nerves contain a mixture of functionally different nerve types: sensory, motor and sympathetic.

Sensory or afferent neurones were discussed in the previous chapter. They transmit signals from periphery to the central nervous system. Nerves in this category are A beta, A delta and C fibres, as discussed in the previous chapter.

Motor or efferent neurones conduct signals from the spinal cord to the muscles. They enable the brain to make muscles contract and control posture and movement. They can be divided into the A alpha and beta motor neurones that innervate muscle fibres and A gamma fibres that control the contractile elements in muscle spindles.

Sympathetic C fibres conduct signals from the central nervous system to effector organs. Strictly speaking, these nerves are efferents, but functionally they are very different from the previous category. Most textbooks focus on the way in which internal organs react in response to sympathetic stimulation, for example increased heart contraction rate or reduced alimentary activity.[1] However, the effects important to the musculoskeletal therapist are in the periphery. For a discussion of these effects, see Chapter 5.

Although cranial nerves originate in the medulla or brain stem rather than the spinal cord, their makeup is similar to peripheral nerves. Pathology of these nerves may give rise to the same symptoms as peripheral neuropathy, as well as symptoms associated with their target organs such as eyes, ears or balance organs.

Note: the parasympathetic nervous system, often described as either the counterpart or the complement of the sympathetic nervous system, is not represented in the peripheral nerves.

Box 3.2 A classic experiment in peripheral neuropathy

Based on Head's experiment, the following stages of uncomplicated nerve recovery can be discerned (Fig. 3.2).[2,3]

Immediately after the lesion there is an area with complete loss of sensation. Around this centre a *hyperpathic* zone develops, an area that feels numb, yet produces unpleasant abnormal sensations when touched with a pin. The skin becomes slightly drier and redder than the surrounding areas (Fig. 3.2.A).

The hyperpathic zone spreads inwards. Numbness is gradually replaced by hypersensitivity, but the centre of the deafferented area remains numb (Fig. 3.2.B). Some cutaneous changes can be observed, such as discoloration or dryness.

The circumference of the hyperpathic zone begins to diminish and sensation in the perimeter gradually returns to normal (Fig. 3.2.C).

By the time the outer zone has regained normal sensitivity, the previously numb centre has become hyperpathic (Fig. 3.2.D).

Finally the centre desensitizes and regains normal sensation. Recovery is complete (Fig. 3.2.E).

In Head's case, the return of normal sensitivity to light touch and temperatures below 37°C took over 500 days.

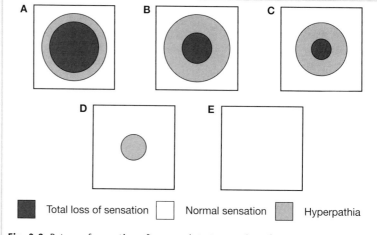

Fig. 3.2 Return of sensation after complete transection of a cutaneous nerve (after [3]).

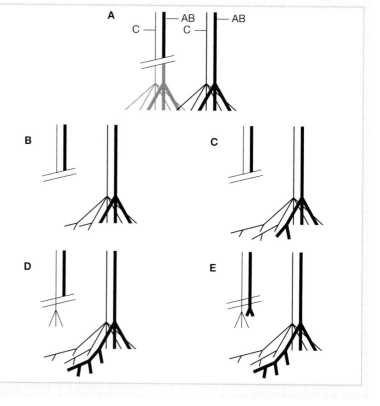

Fig. 3.3 Recovery of C fibres (thin lines) and A beta fibres (thick lines) after transection of a sensory nerve **A**. At first, neighbouring undamaged C fibres sprout **B**, followed by A beta fibres **C**. At a later stage, the damaged nerve itself starts to grow back (**D** and **E**).

The development of hyperpathia in the centre region
(Fig. 3.3.D)

After a while, the proximal end of the transected nerve itself starts to grow back. This is called *direct or regenerative sprouting*. As in collateral sprouting, the unmyelinated fibres penetrate the innervation field first, creating a hyperpathic centre.

Normalization of sensation in the centre (Fig. 3.3.E)

Finally, myelinated fibres from the nerve stump reach the central zone. Eventually the balance of myelinated and unmyelinated nerves is restored in the whole area and sensation returns to normal.

Note: the redness and dryness that Head's colleague observed in the denervated cutaneous region can be explained by a loss of sympathetic innervation.

Head's experiment demonstrates that normal sensation requires both A beta fibres and thinner fibres to be present. The absence of A beta fibres does more than just eradicating the skin's mechanosensitivity, it can actually cause pain. The perception of somatic pain appears to depend on a balance of sensory inputs, rather than purely on nociceptive information. This may be explained by the absence of the moderating influence of the phylogenetically younger A beta fibres described in the previous chapter (Ch. 2, p. 18).

There is compelling evidence that minor neuropathies affecting mainly myelinated fibres may be the reason for non-specific arm pain in office workers.[5,6] This is also known as Repetitive Strain Injury (RSI) or Work Related Upper Limb Disorder (WRULD). It is likely that repeated or sustained force can damage thick afferents.[7] Although the damage may not be sufficient to register on a nerve conduction test, it does create an unbalanced input into the central nervous system.

The importance of the balance of inputs is considered in more detail in Chapter 4. The conclusion that needs to be stressed here is that the manifestation of nerve damage is not restricted to numbness and other classic signs of denervation. *Peripheral neuropathy*, or damage or dysfunction of the peripheral nerve, can manifest in a variety of ways. The rest of this chapter is devoted to these changes and their underlying mechanisms.

PERIPHERAL NEUROGENIC AND NEUROPATHIC PAIN

The current definition of neurogenic pain of the International Association for the Study of Pain is 'Pain initiated or caused by a primary lesion or dysfunction or transitory perturbation in the peripheral or central nervous system.'[8] Neuropathic pain is a sub-category with an almost identical definition: 'Pain initiated or caused by a primary lesion or dysfunction in the peripheral or central nervous system.' In other words, both terms refer to pain as a result of damaged or malfunctioning nerves, but neurogenic pain may be less persistent than neuropathic pain. In practice, the two terms are used interchangeably and refer to pain that is generated in the nervous system. Persistent pain resulting from frank peripheral nerve damage has also been called *causalgia* and is now classed as Complex Regional Pain Syndrome Type 2[9] (see Ch. 5).

The inflammatory process is well defined and initiates fairly predictable mechanisms of pain generation. Appropriate treatment of the algogenic or pain-creating source can be expected to alleviate or eliminate somatic pain. In contrast, the classification, examination and treatment of neurogenic pain are fraught with difficulty.[10–12] Patients may display one or several of a wide range of symptoms, from the obvious to the bizarre. These symptoms may be constant or fluctuate seemingly spontaneously. As a result, patients with neurogenic pains have been classed as 'hysterical' in the past and subjected to inappropriate treatments.

One of the reasons for the complex symptomatology associated with neuropathy, the importance of balance between fibre types, has been discussed already. Matters are complicated by the fact that the nervous system changes its structure and function as a result of dysfunction and damage. This means that persistent neuropathy is associated with changes in signs and symptoms that can be hard to understand. Many patients find it difficult to find a clinician who believes their story, because the symptom behaviour can be very erratic. The clinician who assumes that the pain must be somatic, simply because pain and tenderness manifest in the tissues, may feel that the clinical reasoning process begins to resemble shifting sands. Objective tests are often negative, inconclusive or contradictory, so therapists are forced to rely on subjective descriptions without clear objective markers. This can make it nearly impossible to establish a diagnosis or to rationally assess the effect of a treatment.

In neuropathic pain there is no linear relationship between cause and effect or between pain mechanism and symptom.[13] One mechanism may produce different symptoms in different patients. Conversely, although several patients may describe the same symptoms, these symptoms may be caused by different mechanisms. The difficulty for the clinician is that a mechanism-based treatment can be impossible to find. While inflammatory pain can simply be treated by targeting the underlying mechanism of inflammation, in neuropathic pain the mechanisms are more complex and varied.

Despite these seemingly insurmountable difficulties, there are signs and symptoms that are strongly suggestive of peripheral neuropathy, be it from damage or irritation of a nerve. It may not be possible for the therapist to achieve the same diagnostic certainty as with musculoskeletal conditions. However, knowledge of the genesis, development and manifestations of neurogenic pathology enables him to generate likely hypotheses if a patient fails to respond to treatment. Moreover, it is now thought that many musculoskeletal pains are likely to have a neurogenic component, which may explain why some complaints of a seemingly mechanical nature are refractory to manual and anti-inflammatory therapy. [4-10] The following three sections (pp. 35–38) are devoted to the ways in which neuropathies can manifest, as well as potential underlying mechanisms.

SPONTANEOUS IMPULSE GENERATION

A peculiar property of damaged nerves is that they become capable of generating impulses spontaneously.[4] This is referred to as *ectopic impulse generation*. The word ectopic refers to the fact that the impulse is not generated in the usual way, i.e. by stimulation of the receptors at the peripheral end of the nerve. In sensory research, the resultant pain is referred to as *stimulus-independent pain*, because its development does not rely on stimulation. The neuroma that forms at the proximal end of a damaged nerve, with its high density of fresh nerve endings, is a common origin of ectopic impulses.

These changes along the axon are not always the result of obvious nerve damage. One of the causes of this axonal change is thought to be repeated friction with strong musculoskeletal structures such as fascia or bone.[4] Another cause may be sustained compression. For example, when the median nerve becomes constricted in the carpal tunnel it may begin to generate impulses that give rise to a characteristic tingling sensation in the palm and fingers.

In the areas where a peripheral nerve is subjected to repeated or sustained mechanical force, the nerve's myelin sheath is likely to suffer damage and become a source of ectopic impulse generation.[11] This applies to nociceptive A delta fibres, but also to A beta fibres which normally do not generate pain. In addition, spontaneous C fibre activity has been demonstrated following nerve constriction in animals. For an overview of experimental models of constrictive nerve injuries and conclusions from animal experiments, see Bridges et al.[14]

The mechanism underlying the development of spontaneous impulse generation is a tendency of the nerve to produce increasing numbers of sodium channels in response to damage. These sodium channels are deposited not only in the damaged part of the nerve, but along its entire axon and dorsal root ganglion.[15,16] The reason that the nerve increases its sensitivity in response to nerve damage can be seen as a way of adapting to a loss of input from the periphery (Box 3.3).

In any nerve, the generation of impulses relies on the opening of ion channels (see Ch. 2). When the membrane potential reaches a certain threshold, voltage sensitive sodium channels open, resulting in a barrage of sodium into the nerve cell. In the sensory neurone, this normally happens only when the nerve's receptor is stimulated. However, when another spot along the axon develops a high concentration of sodium channels, that spot becomes very easily excitable. In fact, it may become so excitable that it generates action potentials spontaneously.

It may be clear that the presence of these and other ion channels is not fixed (Fig. 3.4). Ion channels are proteins, which are broken down

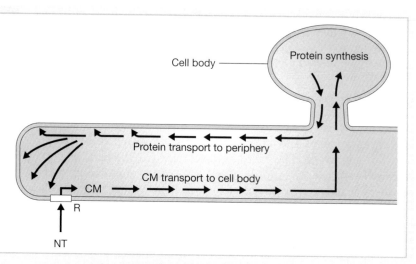

Fig. 3.4 Neurotrophic regulation of the nerve. Tissues produce neurotrophins (NT), which bind with specialized receptors (R) and create reactions inside the nerve cell. Chemical messengers (CM) are transported to the cell body, where they influence the production of proteins. The proteins are transported and deposited along the axon, maintaining or changing the make-up of the nerve.

and replaced continuously just as any other protein in the body. The protein production of a nerve cell takes place in the cell body and is regulated by chemical signals from the tissues that the nerve inner-vates, the so-called *neurotrophic factors*.[16,17] In other words, the production and replacement of ion channels is dependent on contact between the nerve and its target tissue. When a nerve is damaged, the effect of the neurotrophic factors on the activity in the cell body is dis-rupted. In response, the nerve increases the protein production in the cell body, leading to an accumulation of sodium channels along the nerve and considerable increases in excitability. The turnover period of ion channels can be measured in days rather than months, so the adaptation to nerve damage and tissue changes is rapid.[4]

The fact that neuropathic pain can be generated in absence of frank nerve damage has significant implications for manual therapists, because many conditions that are thought of as musculoskeletal or myofascial in origin may in fact be partially or completely neurogenic in nature. The importance of mechanical interfaces between nerves and musculo-skeletal structures has been acknowledged in entrapment syndromes, for instance involving entrapment of the median nerve by the prona-tor teres muscle, or the sciatic nerve by the piriformis muscle.[18] However, there are many other areas where the restriction is less obvi-ous but nonetheless very likely. For instance, it is conceivable that the cutaneous nerves can get trapped where they pierce through the fas-cia in order to get to the skin. This is a potential cause of localized tenderness that mimics musculoskeletal pathology (Fig. 3.5).

RESPONSE TO ACTIVITY IN ADJACENT NERVES

An alternative model explaining spontaneous activity in nociceptive neurones involves so-called *ephaptic* connections. This term refers to the coupling between nerves that normally operate in isolation

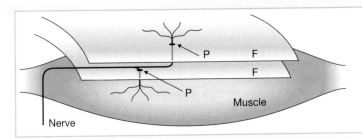

Fig. 3.5 Potential sites for peripheral nerve entrapment potentially leading to myofascial and cutaneous pain. The course of this cutaneous nerve leads it in between sheets of fascia (F), which it has to pierce in order to reach skin or muscle. The nerve is mechanically restricted at passing points (P).

(Fig. 3.6). It can apply to separate nerves, but it is more likely to occur between adjacent nerve fibres within the same peripheral nerve. The nerve's myelin sheath and surrounding connective tissue structure or endoneurium fulfil the role of electrical insulating materials, analogous to the plastic sleeve around electrical wires. Electrical coupling can be thought of as the result of damage to these insulating layers.[4] Ephaptic coupling means that action potentials travelling down the axon of a motor neurone can trigger impulses in sensory nerves where the two are not insulated. If the impulses are generated in nociceptive fibres, the result is an unpleasant sensation. This mechanism has been referred to as *crosstalk*, analogous to the phenomenon of hearing other people's conversation while on the telephone.

Another form of coupling is chemical in nature. Damaged nerves may not just change their production of sodium channels, but also develop receptors for noradrenaline.[19] When local sympathetic nerves are activated they release noradrenaline, which normally does not affect the axon. However, because of the presence of abnormal adrenergic

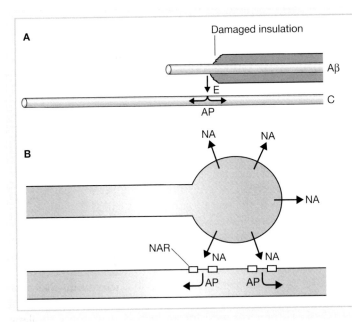

Fig. 3.6 Ephaptic links between low threshold and high threshold nerve fibres. Signals in an A beta fibre with damaged insulation excite (E) an adjacent C fibre, creating action potentials (AP). The release of noradrenaline (NA) triggers action potentials in an adjacent nerve, which has developed noradrenaline receptors (NAR).

receptors, sensory nerves may respond to sympathetic activation. This is discussed in greater detail in Chapter 5.

MECHANOSENSITIVITY

Increased concentrations of sodium channels are not necessarily sufficient for the nerve to become spontaneously active. However, they are likely to make the nerve sensitive to mechanical influences along its axon. The nerves may begin to generate action potentials in response to pressure or stretch, stimuli which normally don't affect them. This gives rise to Tinel's sign, the evocation of sensory symptoms as a result of tapping a nerve, most commonly described for the median nerve as it traverses the carpal tunnel (for example, see [20]). Phalen's test, which involves subjecting the median nerve to sustained pressure, can also identify a neuropathy of the median nerve, as can passive wrist extension.[21] The application of sustained stretch is called the Reversed Phalen's test. Although these types of tests are commonly used on the median nerve, they can in fact be adapted for other peripheral nerves. This was done for the upper limb by Robert Elvey[22] and refined for most of the somatic nervous system by David Butler.[23]

Tests of mechanosensitivity may provoke innocuous but abnormal symptoms such as pins and needles. They may also cause pain, which is then referred to as *stimulus-evoked pain* or *stimulus-dependent pain*.

It is likely that changes along the peripheral nerve are only partially responsible for neuropathic mechanosensitivity. As mentioned before, normal sensation depends on a balanced input from various types of sensory nerve. The input from A beta fibres is important to keep the effect of nociceptive activity under control (please refer to the experiment in Box 3.2). Damage to the myelin sheath of A beta fibres may interfere with their function, thereby reducing their inhibitory function. This phenomenon can be referred to as *disinhibition*.

REDUCTIONS AND INCREASES IN SENSATION

When assessing patients with nerve damage, the observation that is easiest to understand is a reduction in sensation. Stimuli are perceived by the patient, but less strongly than in unaffected areas of the body. The area may even be completely numb. If the stimulus is felt, the modality of the stimulus corresponds with the felt sensation. For example, touch feels like touch, but is perceived as less strong.

A reduction in sensation in general is referred to as *hypoaesthesia*, whereas a reduction in the sensation of pain is called *hypoalgesia*.

The loss or reduction of one sensory modality does not automatically imply the loss of others, so a thorough assessment of a patient with suspected neuropathies should include a range of tactile and thermal stimuli.

The changes in the damaged nerve described above are also likely to lead to an increased response to non-noxious and noxious stimuli. *Hyperaesthesia* is the term used for an increased response to a sensory stimulus. The sub-category *hyperalgesia* refers to an increased response to a stimulus that would be painful even under normal circumstances. Therefore, hyperalgesia refers to a situation where a painful stimulus causes more pain than would normally be expected.

Sometimes a stimulation that would normally not be expected to be painful causes pain. This is referred to as *allodynia*.[24] Neuropathies may engender allodynia in response to one or several types of stimulus. For example, a patient may describe pain in response to gentle mechanical stimuli such as brushing of the skin, but have no allodynia to cold. Cutaneous mechanical allodynia to a dynamic stimulus (stroking) is thought to be mediated by myelinated fibres, whereas a static stimulus (pressure) evokes allodynia by stimulating unmyelinated afferents.[11] Detailed assessment of a patient with suspected neuropathies should always involve a range of modalities (see Examination of neurogenic pain, p. 42).

Patients with peripheral neuropathies may simply have an area of numbness or reduced sensation. This is common after damage of small nerves as a consequence of surgery or injury. Although the lack of sensation can sometimes be a nuisance to the victim, intervention is rarely required. However, in patients suffering pain as a result of nerve damage the situation is more complex. Because various sensory modalities may be affected differentially, patients frequently display a range of seemingly contradictory sensory changes. For example, a patient may find it hard to feel cotton wool dragged across the affected area of skin, but even the gentlest touch with the tip of a needle can cause extreme pain. The following section highlight elements in the patient's history and description suggestive of peripheral neuropathy. This is followed by recommendations regarding assessment.

SUBJECTIVE ASSESSMENT OF NEUROGENIC PAIN

Diagnosing neuropathic pain is not easy. At the annual scientific conference of the British Pain Society in 2004, over 150 professionals specializing in pain were asked whether they felt able to reliably diagnose it. Nobody responded. Nevertheless, the following descriptions in the patient's history are suggestive of a neurogenic origin of pain. If present, these 'neural flags' have to be followed up in the examination of the patient:

- The pain may have started with any form of blunt or sharp trauma, which unfortunately includes surgery (see Scar pain, p. 47). If pain develops immediately or some time after an injury or operation and does not settle over the following months, a neurogenic origin has to be considered. Other potential causes of the pain must be excluded. The pain tends to be either around the site of injury or surgery, but it may also be felt in the innervation area of the peripheral nerve that passes through this site.
- Elements of the patient's history may suggest sustained nerve compression, which can cause temporary or permanent neuropathy. The suggested mechanism is the disruption of local circulation, as

well as the aforementioned local axonal changes. Examples are compression of the common peroneal nerve after sitting cross-legged for a while or radial nerve palsy after sleeping with the arm on the backrest of a seat. Iatrogenic examples are nerve compressions as a result of ill-fitting splints or plaster casts. A haematoma or increase in tissue volume as a result of a clumsy injection may also create increased pressure on a nerve. Pain may radiate more peripherally as time progresses.

- Metabolic problems can interfere with the function of peripheral nerves, for example in diabetes mellitus or vitamin B12 deficiency.[25] Because the causative factor is systemic, the presentation is likely to be symmetrical, although mononeuropathy does occur.[20] The risk of neuropathy increases with the length of nerves, so the lower limbs are most likely to be affected. Several underlying mechanisms have been suggested, such as sensitization of nociceptors, regenerating nerve sprouts and altered activity in the dorsal horn.[26] It is likely that more than one mechanism plays a role in creating the pain. In a recent study of polyneuropathy, the most common pain descriptors were deep aching pain, pain on pressure and pain paroxysms.[26]

- The patient is likely to describe a lack of response to analgesics. Neuropathic pains do not respond to normal analgesics, such as paracetamol and anti-inflammatory drugs. They may even be insensitive to opioids like codeine or morphine.[27]

- The patient may have a history of failed manual treatments. Local mechanical treatments may or may not be of help for neuropathic pain, depending on its target and a variety of factors beyond the therapist's control. It is common for manual therapists to wrongly identify and treat tissue restriction as the source of the pain. For example, pain in response to a muscle stretch may be seen as an indication that the muscle is injured, whereas the real source of pain is a local nerve. It is true that a treatment focused purely on tissue release in the presence of a neuropathy has a chance of reducing the mechanical forces on the nerve, thereby easing the pain. However, because neurogenic changes are associated with mechano-sensitivity, local mechanical treatment may also make the pain worse. Even gentle treatments may stir up symptoms with unexpected intensity. The results of repeated treatments based purely on a tissue-based treatment model are therefore likely to follow a hit and miss pattern.

- Paraesthesia and dysaesthesia are typical of neurogenic pathology. Both terms refer to abnormal sensations, such as pins and needles, running water or crawling ants in absence of such stimuli. The term paraesthesia is used for innocuous sensations. The term dysaesthesia refers to painful sensations, sometimes described as paroxysms of electric shocks.

- Numbness. An area of numbness is the most obvious hint that a nerve may be damaged or not functioning well. Stimuli from the periphery do not reach the brain and are therefore not perceived by the patient. The numbness does not have to be complete. Because often not all nerve types are affected equally by neuropathy, it is possible that a patient feels that the intensity of certain sensations is reduced, whereas others are unaffected or even stronger than normal. A numb area may nevertheless be painful, a phenomenon referred to as *anaesthesia dolorosa*. A damaged sensory nerve can generate pain, which is interpreted by the brain as coming from its normal receptive field. At the same time, stimuli that actually are applied to its cutaneous receptive field are not perceived. These seemingly paradoxical observations sometimes lead patients to doubt their own sanity, thinking that the pain may be 'all in the head'. They may be reluctant to describe all aspects of their pain, unless they are certain that the clinician will accept any description of pain, no matter how extraordinary it may seem.

- Pain resulting from nerve damage is traditionally described as shooting, crushing and burning. However, it manifests in different ways in different patients. In one patient the nature of the pain may change regularly, or a background pain may have paroxysmal shooting pains mixed in. Pain characteristics are likely to change over time as a result of adaptive changes in the peripheral and central nervous system.

  If a clinician limits their palette of diagnostic categories to mechanical and inflammatory syndromes, the changing and unpredictable nature of a patient's pain can easily lead to an exasperating search for the structures at fault. The acknowledgement of the existence of neuropathic pains can simplify the diagnostic process considerably. The variability of the symptoms is no longer confusing. Rather, it is extremely helpful, because it is highly suggestive of a neurogenic element in the generation of pain. Of course the presence of neurogenic symptoms does not exclude co-existing or underlying mechanical pathology, so careful examination and thorough clinical reasoning are essential.

- Patients with neurogenic pain are likely to struggle to find words to describe exactly what they feel. The reason is that neuropathic pain is often different from any normal sensation experienced with the nervous system intact. The quality and behaviour of the symptoms are not like those associated with somatic sensations, even though the brain places them in the body's tissues. It is important that the clinician accepts the patient's inability to express exactly what they are feeling.

  Difficulty in matching a sensation with a description does not indicate lack of intelligence or education, but must be interpreted as a positive indicator that the patient experiences a sensation or sensations that they are utterly unfamiliar with. *It is a mistake to press the patient to give an answer that fits into categories predetermined by the clinician* (burning, shooting, dull, etcetera), because this is likely to yield inaccurate information. Spending an extra minute on the subjective assessment by giving patients the chance to find their own description can save much time later.

- Damaged nerves may develop sensitivity to noradrenaline and adrenaline. Sympathetic nerve fibres secrete noradrenaline, while adrenaline is released into the blood stream by the adrenal glands in response to sympathetic activity. The result can be a pain that increases when the sympathetic nervous system becomes more active, so-called *sympathetically maintained pain*.[13] The sympathetic nervous system responds to a wide range of influences, such as temperature changes, activity levels and emotions, so in some patients neuropathic pain responds to any or all of these factors.

  Some patients describe the sensitivity to sympathetic changes very well, for example by indicating that the pain increases whenever they get cold, or when they feel emotional or generally unwell. Other patients are understandably confused by the seemingly spontaneous changes in their pain, which are independent of their activities. They may say that the behaviour of the pain is completely erratic and may blame their own mental sanity. As with the inability to describe the exact pain sensation, *the clinician has to accept* the patient's inability to identify consistent aggravating and easing factors as positive information, suggestive of neurogenic factors.

- Patients with peripheral neuropathy may describe allodynia or pain caused by innocuous stimuli. Allodynia to touch is most common, followed by allodynia to pressure and cold.[11] Allodynia to warmth is uncommon. In contrast with patients with inflammatory pain, who tend to find cold soothing, some patients with neuropathic pain experience pain when cold is applied. Their pain may also increase when the weather turns cold.

EXAMINATION OF NEUROGENIC PAIN

The aim of the objective examination of the patient with symptoms suggestive of peripheral neuropathy is to find objective evidence for or against the hypothesis. If neurogenic signs are indeed present, the examination should enable the clinician to refine the hypothesis, decide which neural structures are likely to be involved and formulate a rational treatment plan. Once a hypothesis has been formulated, it should be tested in functional ways if possible.

Peripheral nerves contain a mixture of up to three components: sensory, motor and sympathetic. Examination of neuropathy ideally includes all of these, although in practice sensory assessment is easiest to carry out with some detail. An exception to this general rule is the assessment of nerve root pathology, discussed in the following section. Findings must be compared with the opposite side as well as the surrounding area. Care must be taken to apply tests in a consistent way, so that the chance of false positives is minimized.

In the initial examination of any patient, the identification of pathology that requires urgent action is a priority. Signs and symptoms of peripheral neuropathy may be the result of nerve root compression, which may require further investigation and surgical intervention.[28] The diagnosis of nerve root compression is based on changes in sensation, muscle strength and reflexes. These changes should be consistent, i.e. they should all relate to the same segment.

If sensory changes suggestive of nerve root involvement are present, but without corresponding motor changes, other hypotheses have to be considered. Nerve root pain may be the result of chemical irritation of the spinal nerve by material from the nucleus of the intervertebral disc [28-30] rather than an actual entrapment. It is also possible that changes that seem to have their origin in the spinal nerve root stem from a peripheral nerve pathology. For instance, the overlap between the L3 dermatome and the cutaneous region innervated by the femoral nerve necessitate careful examination and clinical reasoning.

The assessment of peripheral neuropathy is based on a thorough knowledge of the anatomy of the peripheral nervous system as well as the cranial nerves. Professionals should be familiar with peripheral neuro-anatomy, but may be advised to consult an anatomy text if a patient presents with symptoms suggestive of neuropathy, especially if they do not follow a clear musculoskeletal pattern. Common entrapment syndromes are discussed below under Specific neuropathies.

Pathology of motor neurones may manifest as muscle weakness, although sometimes muscle fasciculations can be observed.

When the sympathetic fibres of a nerve are affected, the following changes may be observed:

- The sympathetic nerves regulate vasodilation and vasoconstriction, so the affected area may be discoloured and have a different temperature compared with surrounding tissues and the opposite side.
- If circulatory changes persist, tissue quality may suffer. This may manifest as dryness or brittleness of the skin. The soft tissues may demonstrate an increased resistance to stretch as a result of ongoing trophic changes.
- Sudomotor activity is under direct control of the sympathetic nerves. The affected area may be either drier or sweatier than comparable cutaneous regions.
- Pilo erection is a sympathetic phenomenon. The hairs in the area innervated by the affected nerve may stand on end, either spontaneously or in response to cutaneous stimulation.
- Cranial nerves are involved in non-cutaneous aspects of autonomic regulation, such as dilation of the pupils.

  Because neuropathy affects the various sensory modalities in different ways, it is important to test more than one modality.

- Light touch can be tested with cotton wool or a small thin-haired brush. Make sure that the contact area, pressure applied, and length and timing of the stroke are consistent.
- Sensitivity to sharpness is tested by touching the skin with the tip of a needle such as a needle used for injections or acupuncture, or a neurotip. Consistency can be improved by using an aesthesiometer or pinwheel, using the weight of the instrument to control pressure (Fig. 3.7.A). In effect, this instrument consists of series of neurotips that can be applied in quick succession.

Fig. 3.7 Instruments used for sensory testing in the clinic. **A.** The aesthesiometer. **B.** The Lindblom roller.

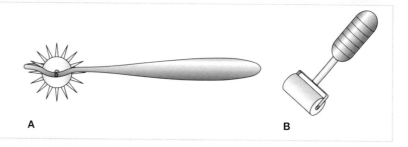

A   B

- Sensitivity to coolness can be tested with a metal roller, for example made of aluminium, with a handle to avoid warming by the examiner (Fig. 3.7.B).[31] The roller can be kept at room temperature or lower. Accuracy is improved if the exact temperature is recorded and maintained when further tests are done. The advantage of the roller over the traditional test tube is that a wide area can be investigated without having to lift and lower the instrument repeatedly and without moving it across the skin.

- Sensitivity to warmth can be investigated by keeping a metal roller at a certain temperature by placing it in a baby bottle warmer. In practice, a temperature of 40 °C is adequate (see for instance [32,33] for more detailed information).

- Myelinated afferents can be tested selectively using vibration. This is particularly useful if the patient's symptoms are suggestive of a neuropathy, but other clinical tests fail to elicit them. Unfortunately, at present vibration is not easy to test in the clinical environment. The most common method involves putting a tuning fork on the skin, which carries inherent sources of error such as the lack of control over the amplitude of the vibration and the pressure of application. The use of a calibrated electronic vibrometer is recommended.

- A mixture of hypoaesthesia and hyperaesthesia is typical of neuropathy. For example, the patient may hardly feel that an area of skin is touched with cotton wool. However, if the same area is touched with the tip of a needle, it may cause acute pain. This is an example of the paradoxical nature of neurogenic pain. Therefore, sensory testing should involve at least light touch and pinprick.

- Sensory changes may be limited to sensitivity to temperature if only thin nerve fibres are affected.[11] If sensitivity to touch is normal but the clinician has a strong suspicion of neuropathy, tests of sensitivity to warmth and coolness can be added.

- Tinel's test involves tapping a peripheral nerve, in order to assess whether it is mechanosensitive.[20] The test is regarded positive if it elicits sensations distal to the stimulation site, such as paraesthesia or pain. It is commonly used in the assessment of suspected carpal tunnel syndrome, but it can be applied anywhere along a peripheral nerve. Normally, a peripheral nerve is not sensitive to mechanical stimulation along its axon. However, when mechanical constriction leads to the generation of ectopic impulse generating sites, percussion can generate symptoms.[4]

- Sometimes nerve compression for 90 seconds is used to test peripheral nerve compression. Examples of the application of compression are sustained end of range wrist flexion in testing the carpal tunnel (Phalen's test), or Wright's test to investigate compression sensitivity of the brachial plexus.[21]
- Palpation can identify sites of mechanosensitivity of peripheral sensory nerves.[23] Robert Maigne points out that pain from the nerves originating at the thoracolumbar junction can easily be mistaken for pain of lumbosacral origin.[34] He recommends the palpation of these nerves as they traverse the posterior ilium with the patient in flexion as one of the ways of assessing their involvement. The ilio-inguinal and genitofemoral nerves may need to be assessed when a patient presents with pain in the groin and anterior thigh (Fig. 3.8).

Doctors may request electrical nerve conduction studies, to see whether and where there is an interruption in continuity of peripheral nerves. However, these tests will only be positive if the disruption of the bundle of nerves is considerable. The number of fibres left intact in nerves with only minor or moderate damage may conduct all of the current. Nerve fibres run parallel to one another; a few damaged fibres do not affect the conduction of the whole nerve (Fig. 3.9). In other words, if the test is positive the damage is beyond doubt, but *a lack of findings does not exclude it.*

If the patient has a history of abdominal surgery, the following test can demonstrate whether the pain is likely to be of visceral origin, or the result of nerve entrapment in the abdominal wall. The patient lies supine. The painful area is palpated so that the pain is reproduced.

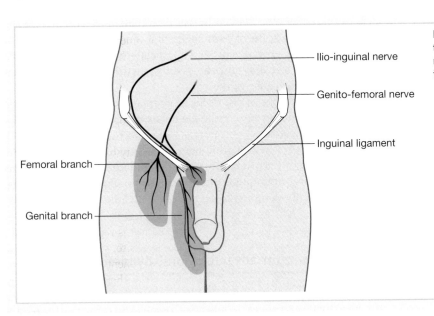

Fig. 3.8 The course followed by the ilio-inguinal and genitofemoral nerves and their cutaneous innervation area (based on [54,55]).

Ilio-inguinal nerve

Genito-femoral nerve

Inguinal ligament

Femoral branch

Genital branch

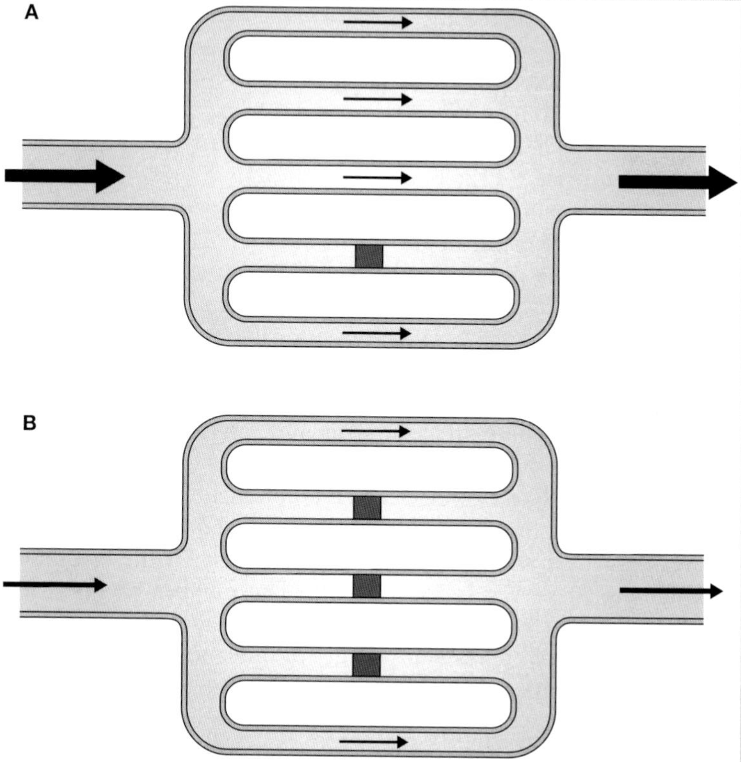

Fig. 3.9 The electrical conduction through a bundle of nerve fibres is analogous to the flow of water through a set of parallel pipes. **A.** Obstruction of one pipe leaves other pipes to maintain the flow. **B.** Only the obstruction of a large proportion of parallel channels increases the resistance appreciably, thereby reducing the flow.

Next, the patient is asked to lift their head off the couch, which causes the abdominal muscles to tense. If the palpation pain has a visceral origin, it is likely to reduce, because the increased abdominal muscle tension reduces the manual pressure on the affected organ. On the other hand, an increase in pain suggests a more superficial origin of pain, making an entrapment of superficial nerves more likely. Be aware that this test may also be positive if the abdominal muscles themselves are the cause of the pain.

As always, this type of test needs to be treated with caution. If there is any doubt whatsoever over the diagnosis of abdominal pain, a doctor must be consulted.

The diagnosis of neuropathic pain may be aided by the use of the Leeds assessment of neuropathic symptoms and signs (LANSS).[35] This tool consists of a brief questionnaire and some simple objective tests. It was specifically designed to be used in the clinic as opposed to the laboratory.

A critical note on adverse neural dynamics

David Butler's original model of adverse neural tension was based on the idea that nerves were connective tissue structures that needed a certain degree of mobility in order to function well.[23] He reasoned that nerves passed through a number of mechanical interfaces, for instance the exit foramen of the spine, the thoracic outlet or certain muscle groups, and that these structures could interfere with their passage. Examination and treatment focused on areas of neural tethering, which could be found by putting a nerve under tension.

It seems more likely that the assessment of neural tension in fact demonstrates the presence or absence of mechanosensitivity of the nerve. Neural changes are most likely at places where the nerve is mechanically restricted,[4] hence the pain and apparent resistance to movement of the nerve in those areas. To his credit, Butler has revised his original views and integrated them in a greater and more realistic perspective.[36]

SPECIFIC NEUROPATHIES

The discussion of every neuropathic pain syndrome is beyond the scope of this book; however, some of these syndromes tend not to be addressed in clinical texts for musculoskeletal practitioners, even though they occur commonly. As a result they frequently remain unrecognized and therefore treated wrongly, if they are treated at all. An additional reason for their inclusion in this chapter is that they give an idea of the range of manifestations of persistent neuropathic pain.

Scar pain

A common but under-acknowledged form of neuropathic pain is pain following surgery. In a study of more than 5000 patients, over 20% had pain as a result of surgical intervention.[37] Even operations that leave only small scars such as vasectomies and hernia repairs, have a high incidence of post-surgical pain. In stark contrast with these statistics, surgical textbooks make little mention of its occurrence, or state that neuralgias can be expected to resolve within days to weeks after the operation.[38]

Post-surgical pain can easily be misinterpreted and therefore go untreated. Pain at initial review following surgery is likely to be seen as part of the recovery process. If the pain remains, the specialist may try to determine whether there is a problem with the organ or structure that was operated on, or whether there is additional pathology. For example, physical examination and an abdominal ultrasound scan may be repeated following gynaecological surgery. If the examination and further tests do not establish a cause for the pain, the surgeon is likely to conclude that the operation was successful and that there is no suggestion of complication or additional pathology. In other words, the patient may feel pain, but its resolution is no longer the responsibility of the specialist. The patient may be discharged, or referred on to a pain clinic or a therapist.

A young man, 30 years of age, had surgery because of a benign fatty growth in the right breast area. After the operation, he developed a pain around the scar. Over the months, this pain intensified. It started to spread to his flank, and from there to his scapula and back. It also spread upwards to his upper trapezius region and down into his arm. The physiotherapist established that a restriction in the mobility of the scar contributed to the pain. This was demonstrated by the fact that shoulder flexion caused widespread pain, unless the skin around the scar was supported and lifted. Treatment of the mobility of the scar and surrounding superficial soft tissues reduced the spread of pain, until after a few months it was felt over the scar only.

The mechanism responsible for post-surgical pain is thought to be the nerve damage caused by the surgical incision, for example in the case described in Box 3.4. After surgery, transected nerves begin to repair. Usually this is uneventful, perhaps leaving a small area of cutaneous numbness. However, regenerating nerve fibres may get caught in the scar tissue, which tightens as it matures. Alternatively, scar tissue may prevent recovering nerve fibres from reaching their original target area. The latter is particularly pertinent to the recovery of myelinated fibres, which have to find their myelin sheaths following nerve injury.[3,39] Whatever the exact mechanism, both neural constriction and the formation of neuromas as a result of incomplete recovery is likely to lead to the onset of neuropathic pain that can be extremely resistant to treatment.[4]

When assessing a patient with pain that may be associated with surgery, it is essential that potential pathology is excluded. If there is any suspicion that an infection or malignancy is present, the patient's General Practitioner or specialist must be consulted. The same applies when thorough examination and clinical reasoning leave question marks regarding the origin of the pain. Pain must never be treated in its own right, unless either the underlying pathology has been identified or it is certain that the pain is not the result of pathology. If the patient underwent surgery for cancer, this is especially pertinent. In particular, cancer pain that returns after a pain free period must be treated with suspicion.

An additional reason for a referral to a medical practitioner is a patient's fear about stitches that were left in by mistake, or surgical instruments that were not taken out. Reassurances that do not seem genuine and well founded to the patient are likely to raise anxiety and may lead to ideas of conspiracy. A patient who is fearful regarding post-surgical complications is not in a position to focus on managing the pain, as will be explained in Chapters 6 and 7.

Manual therapists are familiar with the peripheral nerves innervating the limbs. Of specific importance for post-surgical pain is the course followed by the thoracic and abdominal nerves. Specifically, the genitofemoral and ilioinguinal nerves (Fig. 3.8) can easily be damaged by vasectomy, sterilization or caesarian section. Other forms of blunt or sharp trauma may also damage these nerves, so trunk injuries unresponsive to physical therapy warrant a sensory assessment. Finally, nerve root pathology must be considered if sensory tests are positive.

Thoracic outlet syndrome

The brachial plexus has to pass through three potentially restrictive openings before it reaches the upper limb.[18] First it passes between the anterior and intermediate scalenus muscles. This passageway can be tested with Adson's test. Next, it runs between the clavicle and the first rib, examined in Eden's test and Roos' test. Finally, it passes under the pectoralis minor muscle. Restriction here is assessed by applying Wright's test, also called the hyperabduction test. Thoracic outlet syndrome is less specific than entrapment of a single nerve root or peripheral nerve, so it can be more difficult to recognize.

Table 3.1 Entrapment neuropathies of the extremities

Nerve	Entrapment site	Symptoms	May masquerade as
Radial	Lateral elbow	Pain and sensory changes radial distribution	Tennis elbow, De Quervain's
Median	Carpal tunnel	Paraesthesia and pain hand	–
Median	Pronator teres	Pain in median distribution	Carpal tunnel syndrome
Ulnar	Cubital tunnel	Pain and sensory changes ulnar distribution	–
Ulnar	Tunnel of Guyon	Pain and sensory changes ulnar distribution	–
Lateral femoral cutaneous	Inguinal ligament	Pain and sensory changes anterolateral thigh	L3 nerve root entrapment
Saphenus	Medial knee	Medial knee and calf pain	–
Common peroneal	Proximal fibular head	Pain and sensory changes anterolateral lower leg & dorsum foot	L4–5 nerve root entrapment
Superficial peroneal	Lateral lower leg	Pain and sensory changes dorsum foot and first four toes	L5 nerve root entrapment
Deep peroneal	Metatarsal 1	Pain first and second toe	–
Tibial	Medial ankle (tarsal tunnel)	Pain heel, sole and toes	L5–S1 nerve root entrapment
Medial and lateral plantar	Medial calcaneum	Pain sole and toes	Plantar faciitis, tibialis posterior tendonitis, tarsal tunnel syndrome
Digital pedal	Between metatarsal heads	Pain in toe, typically 3rd or 4th	–

Entrapment neuropathies

Peripheral nerves pass through narrow areas, where they can be mechanically compromised. Table 3.1 gives an overview.[18]

Overuse injuries of the upper limb

Pain as a result of repetitive movements carried out over a long period has been a mystery for many years. It has been called repetitive strain injury (RSI), work-related upper limb disorder (WRULD) and non-specific arm pain (NSAP), and is prevalent in factory workers, users of computer keyboards and musicians. The pain can manifest in many ways and can be extremely unpredictable. Therapists jumping to conclusions about the patient's mental state only demonstrate their own ignorance.

Studies by Lynn and Greening[6,40,41] suggest that these overuse injuries are likely to be associated with minor neuropathies. The lack of variety in posture and type of movement in office workers may create a constriction of peripheral nerves that generates neural changes over time. The resultant pain is often mistakenly interpreted as a sign of pathology of the musculoskeletal structures close to the nerve. For example, as mentioned in Table 3.1 the manifestation of radial neuropathy may be very similar to lateral epicondylitis or De Quervain's, but any benefits from treatment using local injections and manual therapy are unlikely to last if the pain is neurogenic in nature.

Episacro-iliac lipoma

Grieve describes his experience with the benign accumulation of fatty tissue surrounding a nerve overlying the posterior ilium and sacrum.[42] This can generate symptoms very similar to sacro-iliac dysfunction and often the patient has a history of failed investigations and treatments. In this author's experience, on palpation the lipoma can manifest as a soft, mobile lump or as stringy gristle overlying the sacro-iliac sulcus. Grieve recommends injection with local anaesthetic or, if necessary, radiofrequency lesioning of the nerve. The latter can be carried out by anaesthetists in pain clinics, but it may be necessary to give them a clear and detailed explanation of what is required.

TREATMENT OPTIONS

Approaches to the management of neuropathic pain should be based on knowledge of its causative mechanisms. Too often is treatment applied to a musculoskeletal structure simply because it seems to cause pain. However, based on the discussion of mechanisms of neuropathic pain, current treatment methods can be classified as follows:

- The reduction of mechanical constriction of the peripheral nerve. This means that a mechanical model is applied with a neural model in mind.

- The facilitation of neural recovery after injury.
- Blocking sodium channels. This is done chemically, i.e. by the administration of drugs, either orally or via injection.
- Maximizing normal input into the dorsal horn and minimizing nociceptive stimulation. This is the subject of Chapter 4.
- Maximizing the influence of the mind and descending inhibition of pain, which is discussed in Chapter 7.

In layman's terms, these methods could be summarized as 'being nice' to nerves.

In practice, the following treatment approaches are recommended. Some of these methods are more evidence-backed than others.

As with all pain syndromes, it is essential that the patient gains insight into the origin and behaviour of the pain. This reduces the uncertainty and stress associated with the pain, establishes realistic expectations and inspires confidence. The patient should understand the principles on which the suggested treatment is based and be aware of potential side-effects and complications.

The description of the nerves as signalling wires, an analogy used at the beginning of this chapter, can clarify contradictory symptoms such as pain in a numb area. Many patients find the analogy easier to follow if it is drawn for them on a sheet of paper. The mechanism of nerve constriction and its manual release requires the explanation of mechanical interfaces of the nerve. Clinicians who feel that their drawing skills are inadequate may find it helpful to collect drawings from books or colleagues in a folder.

Nerves recover slowly in comparison with muscles and bones, especially when the cytoskeleton of the axon has been damaged. Proteins needed for the reconstruction of damaged nerves are transported from cell body to the periphery by the so-called *slow axonal transport* of up to 2.5 mm per day.[43] An estimate of the distance between the spinal origin of a nerve and the site of injury will give the clinician some idea of the minimum time it will take the first proteins to arrive where they are needed.

If the sciatic nerve suffers degenerative changes as a result of a nerve root entrapment, decompressing surgery or another form of resolution is only the start of the neural recovery process. It is instructive to measure the distance from spine to foot and calculate how long it takes for proteins to travel along the sciatic nerve. It is important to make patients aware of this slow recovery process, because it gives them a realistic expectation. The patient who thinks that the nerve pain should resolve soon after the compression is resolved may visit clinic after clinic in search of a non-existent cure. There is however a place for treatment that focuses on creating optimal circumstances for recovery, for instance by maintaining mobility and updating exercises and advice from time to time. Because the recovery process is slow, the occasional 'maintenance' visit may be all that is required.

Nerve stimulation therapy is sometimes beneficial. Acupuncture is a form of nerve stimulation, as is Transcutaneous Electrical Nerve Stimulation (TENS) and an ever-expanding list of other electrical

A female patient in her 50s presented at a pain clinic for post-surgical pain. Thirteen years earlier, she had undergone surgery to remove her gallbladder and had suffered with pain and hypersensitivity since. The pain kept her awake. The area medial to the scar was so sensitive to light touch that she was unable to wear a bra. Even the brushing of very loose clothes against her skin caused extreme discomfort.

The therapist in the pain clinic did not expect much from a TENS machine after so many years. Much to his surprise and the patient's delight, the use of TENS for 20 min three times per day reduced the symptoms to a minimum within 2 weeks.

modalities. TENS may be the most appropriate option, because its size and cost allows for a patient to use it whenever necessary. The mechanisms and manifestations of neuropathic pain are extremely varied, so it is most beneficial to ignore contradictory and conflicting research about exact stimulation frequencies and doses[44,45] and encourage the patient to experiment.

While in some cases stimulation therapy works extremely well (see Box 3.5 for an example from the author's experience), in others the results may be disappointing. Some patients find that electrical stimulation irritates the site, possibly because of allodynia. However, a sensible trial of nerve stimulation is unlikely to have lasting detrimental effects. Clinicians are referred to appropriate literature for more specific advice, for example by Walsh.[46]

Another form of stimulation therapy is a desensitizing regime that the patient can follow at home. The patient is asked to rub the affected area regularly, starting with a light material such as cotton wool. As the response to this form of touch decreases, a material that offers more friction is chosen, such as a soft towel, then a rough towel, etc. This method sometimes helps to reduce hyperaesthesia, but it is potentially counterproductive if touch allodynia is present.

Empirically, soft tissue techniques such as Myofascial Release and Connective Tissue Manipulation can be effective for scar pain. The myofascial model used by both approaches proposes that the body's soft tissues are layered in sheets of skin, superficial fascia and deep fascia.[47] Scar tissue is seen as reducing the glide between these layers, increasing the mechanical force on local nerves when the tissues are stretched. Restoration of glide and mobility can sometimes have dramatic effects on scar pain, as illustrated by the example in Box 3.5.

The benefits of injection with local anaesthetic are frequently short-lived, although they are sometimes capable of 'resetting' the nerve. Even if the effects don't last, injections can be extremely useful in conjunction with manual therapy. For example, a therapist may suspect that a soft tissue restriction is an important factor in the maintenance of a peripheral neurogenic pain. Treatment of this restriction may cause unacceptable levels of pain, but an injection may create a window of opportunity. Naturally, close cooperation between the treatments of physician and manual therapist are essential for the success of this approach.

Tricyclic anti-depressant drugs have a number of effects on ion channels and receptors that can help to reduce neuropathic pain,[48] although the exact mechanism of action is not certain. [49] The best-known drug is amitriptyline, which can be taken at a 10 or 25 mg to avoid antidepressant effects. If taken at night, the side effect of drowsiness can be an advantage and is likely to have worn off in the morning. When recommending an anti-depressant drug for pain control, it is important that the patient understands that depression is not the reason for the presciption, but that the drug has other non-psychological effects when taken at a low dose. The analgesic effects take a couple of weeks to build up and during that period any side effects are likely to reduce. However, to some patients the side effects are of an unacceptable level. A useful overview of the efficacy of tricyclics and other drugs for neuropathic pain is provided by Kingery.[49]

Anticonvulsant drugs may also be useful for neuropathic pain. Although the assumption that both convulsions and neuropathic pain are the result of excessive neural activity is appealing, the exact mode of action is not clear.[50] Carbamazepine is used mostly for trigeminal neuralgia.[50,51] Gabapentin has been shown to provide relief for post-herpetic neuralgia and diabetic neuropathy.[51,52] Generally, it is tolerated well by patients.

Although NSAIDs are unlikely to affect neuropathic pain, they may be of benefit if an ongoing inflammatory process coexists with a neuropathy. The combination of an NSAID with a so-called *adjuvant drug* like amitriptyline or gabapentin may be more effective than the use of one drug on its own. Similarly, manual therapy and the prescription of adjuvant drugs can be mutually beneficial.

Treatment effectiveness can be difficult to evaluate for neuropathic pain. Recently the Neuropathic Pain Symptom Inventory, a validated questionnaire for the assessment of the 10 most salient symptoms was developed for this purpose.[53]

References

[1] Guyton A, Hall J. Textbook of medical physiology. Philadelphia: WB Saunders, 2000

[2] Rivers W, Head H. A human experiment in nerve division. In: Head H, ed. Studies in neurology. London: Frowde, Hodder & Stoughton, 1920: 225–329

[3] Bernards A. Perifere zenuw laesies. Arnhem: Hogeschool Interstudie, 1987

[4] Devor M, Seltzer Z. Pathophysiology of damaged nerves in relation to chronic pain. In: Wall P, ed. Textbook of pain. 1999: 129–164

[5] Greening J, Lynn B. Vibration sense in the upper limb in patients with repetitive strain injury and a group of at-risk office workers. International Archives of Occupational and Environmental Health 1998; 71:29–34

[6] Greening J, Lynn B, Leary R. Sensory and autonomic function in the hands of patients with non-specific arm pain (NSAP) and asymptomatic office workers. Pain 2003; 104(1,2): 275–282

[7] Gracely R, Lynch S, Bennett G. Painful neuropathy: altered central processing maintained dynamically by peripheral input. Pain 1992; 51:175–194

[8] Merskey H, Bogduk N. Classification of chronic pain. Descriptions of chronic pain syndromes and definitions of pain terms, 2nd edn. Seattle: IASP Press 1994

[9] Boas R. Complex Regional pain syndromes: symptoms, signs, and differential diagnosis. In: Stanton-Hicks M, Jänig W, eds. Reflex sympathetic dystrophy: a reappraisal. Seattle: IASP Press 1996: 79–92

[10] Jensen T, Baron R. Translation of symptoms and signs into mechanisms in neuropathic pain. Pain 2003; 102(1,2):1–8

[12] Hansson P, Kinnman E. Unmasking mechanisms of peripheral neuropathic pain in a clinical perspective. Pain Rev 1996; 3(4):272–292

[12] Hansson P. Difficulties in stratifying neuropathic pain by mechanisms. Eur J Pain 2003; 7(4):353–358

CONCLUSION

Patients may present with symptoms that are not entirely consistent within a tissue-focused clinical reasoning model, but that can be explained by functional and structural peripheral nerve changes. The diagnosis of neuropathic pain presents the clinician with considerable challenges. Symptoms vary considerably per patient and can be subject to unpredictable change within the individual. Objective signs are easily missed unless they are sought deliberately. Finally, where peripheral nerves run concurrent with musculoskeletal tissues, their pathologies can be hard to distinguish from each other.

Mechanical treatments have their place in the management of neuropathic pain, especially in improving mechanical circumstances for the peripheral nerves. A prerequisite is that the clinician makes a decision to treat soft tissues to improve neural pathomechanics rather than the tissues themselves. Neuropathic pain is a diagnostic and therapeutic challenge for patients, scientists and clinicians, but an understanding of potential mechanisms can avoid much frustration in the clinic. By combining advice, exercise, ergonomics, manual therapy, stimulation therapy and the appropriate medical interventions, the patient is given an optimum chance to achieve control over the pain.

For reasons of clarity, this chapter has focused on changes in and treatments of the peripheral nerve. In reality, both persistent inflammatory and neuropathic pains can lead to changes in the central nervous system, which are likely to modify pain perception. These changes are the subject of the following chapter.

[13] Woolf C, Mannion R. Neuropathic pain: aetiology, symptoms, mechanisms, and management. Lancet 1999; 353:1959–1964

[14] Bridges D, Thompson S, Rice A. Mechanisms of neuropathic pain. Br J Anaesth 2001; 87(1):12–26

[15] Devor M, Lomazov P, Matzner O. Sodium channel accumulation in injured axons as a substrate for neuropathic pain. In: Boivie J, Hansson P, Lindblom U, eds. Touch, temperature, and pain in health and disease: mechanisms and assessment. Seattle: IASP Press 1994: 207–230

[16] Black J, Dib-Hajj S, Cummins T, et al. Sodium channels as therapeutic targets in neuropathic pain. In: Hansson P, Fields H, Hill R, Marchetti P, eds. Neuropathic pain: pathophysiology and treatment. Seattle: IASP Press 2002: 19–36

[17] Jessell T, Sanes J. The generation and survival of nerve cells. In: Kandel E, Schwartz J, Jessell T, eds. Principles of neural science. New York, McGraw-Hill, 2000: 1041–1062

[18] Winkel D, Fisher S, Vroege C. Weke delen aandoeningen van het bewegingsapparaat (Soft tissue pathology of the musculoskeletal system). Deel 2: Diagnostiek. Utrecht, Bohn, Scheltema and Holkema 1984

[19] Jänig W, Baron R. The role of the sympathetic nervous system in neuropathic pain: clinical observations and animal models. In: Hansson P, Fields H, Hill R, Marchetti P, eds. Neuropathic pain: pathophysiology and treatment. Seattle: IASP Press 2002: 125–149

[20] Clarke C. Neurological disease. In: Kumar P, Clark M, eds. Clinical medicine. Edinburgh: Saunders 2002: 1123–1224

[21] Magee D. Orthopedic physical assessment, 4th edn. Philadelphia: Saunders, 2002

[22] Kennealy M, Rubenach H, Elvey R. The upper limb tension test: the SLR test of the arm. In: Grant R, ed. Physical therapy of the cervical and thoracic spine. New York: Churchill Livingstone 1988: 167–194

[23] Butler D. Mobilisation of the nervous system. Melbourne: Churchill Livingstone, 1991

[24] Ochoa J. Quantifying sensation: 'Look back in allodynia'. Eur J Pain 2003; 7(4):369–374

[25] Rowland L. Diseases of the motor unit. In: Kandel E, Schwartz J, Jessell T, eds. Principles of neural science. New York: McGraw Hill, 2000: 695–712

[26] Otto M, Bak S, Bach F, Jensen T, Sindrup S. Pain phenomena and possible mechanisms in patients with painful polyneuropathy. Pain 2003; 101(1,2):187–192

[27] Rowbotham M. Efficacy of opioids in neuropathic pain. In: Hansson P, Fields H, Hill R, Marchetti P, eds. Neuropathic pain: pathophysiology and treatment. Seattle: IASP Press 2002: 203–213

[29] Clinical Standards Advisory Group. CSAG Report on low back pain. 1994, 1–89

[29] Olmarker K, Rydevik B, Nordborg C. Autologous nucleus pulposus induces neurophysiologic and histologic changes in porcine cauda equina nerve roots. Spine 1993; 18(11):1425–1432

[30] Obata K, Tsujino H, Yamanaka H, Yi D, Fukuoka T, Hashimoto N, et al. Expression of neurotrophic factors in the dorsal root ganglion in a rat model of lumbar disc herniation. Pain 2002; 99(1,2):121–132.

[31] Marchetti P, Marangonic C, Lacerenza M, Formaglio F. The Lindblom roller. Eur J Pain 2003; 7(4):359–364

[32] Lindblom U. Analysis of abnormal touch, pain and temperature sensation in patients. In: Boivie J, Hansson P, Lindblom U, eds. Touch, temperature and pain in health and disease. Seattle: IASP Press, 1994: 63–84

[33] Hansson P. Possibilities and potential pitfalls of combined bedside and quantitative somatosensory analysis in pain patients. In: Boivie J, Hansson P, Lindblom U, eds. Touch, temperature, and pain in health and disease: mechanisms and assessments. Seattle: IASP Press, 1994:113–132

[34] Maigne R. Low back pain of thoracolumbar origin. Archives of Physical Medicine and Rehabilitation 1980; 61(September):389–394

[35] Bennett P. The LANSS pain scale: the Leeds assessment of neuropathic symptoms and signs. Pain 2001; 92(1,2):147–158

[36] Butler D. The sensitive nervous system. Adelaide: NOI Publications 2000

[37] Crombie I, Davies H, Macrae W. Cut and thrust: antecedent surgery and trauma among patients attending a chronic pain clinic. Pain 1998; 76(1,2):167–172

[38] Macrae W, Davies H. Chronic post-surgical pain. In: Crombie I, ed. Epidemiology of pain. Seattle: IASP Press 1999

[39] Sanes J, Jessell T. The formation and regeneration of synapses. In: Kandel E, Schwartz J, Jessell T, eds. Principles of neural science. New York: McGraw-Hill 2000: 1087–1114

[40] Greening J, Lynn B. Minor peripheral nerve injuries: an underestimated source of pain? Man Ther 1998; 3(4):187–194

[41] Greening J, Smart S, Leary R, Hall-Craggs M, Lynn B. Reduced movement of the median nerve in carpal tunnel during wrist flexion in patients with non-specific arm pain. Lancet 1999; 354:217–218

[42] Grieve G. Episacroiliac lipoma. Physiotherapy 1990; 76(6):308–310

[43] Schwartz J, De Camilli P. Synthesis and trafficking of neuronal proteins. In: Kandel E, Schwartz J, Jessell T, eds. Principles of neural science. New York: McGraw-Hill 2000: 88–104

[44] Johnson M. Acupuncture-like transcutaneous electrical nerve stimulation (AL-TENS) in the management of pain. Physical Therapy Reviews 1998; 3:73–93

[45] Johnson M. A critical review of the analgesic effects of TENS-like devices. Physical Therapy Reviews 2001; 6(3):1–21

[46] Walsh D. TENS. Clinical applications and related theory, 1st edn. New York: Churchill Livingstone, 1997

[47] Manheim C. The myofascial release manual, 2nd edn. Thorofare, NJ: SLACK, 1994

[48] Sindrup S, Jensen T. Antidepressants in the treatment of neuropathic pain. In: Hansson P, Fields H, Hill R, Marchetti P, eds. Neuropathic pain: pathophysiology and treatment. Seattle: IASP Press 2002: 169–183

[49] Kingery W. A critical review of controlled clinical trials for peripheral neuropathic pain and complex regional pain syndromes. Pain 1997; 73(2):123–139

[50] Berde C. New and old anticonvulsants for management of pain. IASP Newsletter 1997;3–6

[51] Backonja M. Anticonvulsants and antiarrhythmics in the treatment of neuropathic pain syndromes. In: Hansson P, Fields H, Hill R, Marchetti P, eds. Neuropathic pain: pathophysiology and treatment. Seattle: IASP Press 2002: 185–201

[52] Rowbotham M, Harden N, Stacey B, Bernstein P, Magnus-Miller L. Gabapentin for the treatment of postherpetic neuralgia. Journal of the American Medical Association 1998; 280(21):1837–1842

[53] Bouhassira D, Attal N, Fermanian J, et al. Development and validation of the Neuropathic Pain Symptom Inventory. Pain 2004; 108(3):248–257

[54] Brown D. Atlas of regional anesthesia, 2 edn. Philadelphia: WB Saunders 1998

[55] Ferner H, Staubesand J. Sobotta atlas of human anatomy, 10th edn. München, Urban and Schwartzenberg, 1982

A selfish switchboard: the dorsal horn

I could tell you how many steps make up the streets rising like stairways, and the degree of the arcades' curves, and what kind of zinc scales cover the roofs; but I already know this would be the same as telling you nothing.

ITALO CALVINO, INVISIBLE CITIES

INTRODUCTION

Sensory information enters the central nervous system in the dorsal horn, from where it is passed up the spinal cord to the brain. The dorsal horn used to be thought of simply as a relay station, which transferred the signals corresponding with each type of sensation on to its own dedicated tract.

It is now clear that although the impulses produced by each type of sensation are passed on through dedicated pathways to a certain degree, the dorsal horn has the capacity to filter, modify and integrate them. The dorsal horn can therefore be conceptualized as a switchboard with an attitude. Sensations including pain can be amplified or attenuated, pains from visceral and somatic structures can get mixed up and innocuous stimuli can increase pain. If the dorsal horn had a passive function and if nociception and non-noxious perception were completely separate, these phenomena would be impossible.

Weighing up a variety of factors, the central nervous system makes an active decision about how incoming peripheral information is processed. To a large extent, this decision is made in the brain but implemented in the dorsal horn (see Ch. 7). The processing state of the dorsal horn determines whether and how pain is perceived. It can suppress incoming information, put it under a magnifying glass, or process it relatively unchanged. The result of this active intervention is that the exact nature of sensory perception does not have a consistent relationship with a stimulus.

This chapter discusses how the dorsal horn can change the way pain is perceived. It explains how mild stimuli such as massage or TENS can *relieve* pain under some circumstances, but can *cause* pain in others. The physiology underlying these processes is complex and not completely understood, but an attempt is made to demonstrate how neural systems make the dorsal horn the adaptive centre that it is.

Box 4.1 Signal transmission in the synapse

The junction of two neurones is called a synapse, a term coined by the British neurologist Sherrington just before the beginning of the 20th century.[1] At the synapse, an electrical signal (the action potential reaching the terminal of a nerve) is converted into a chemical signal (Fig. 4.3). When an action potential reaches the final part of the nerve, the *presynaptic membrane*, voltage sensitive calcium channels open up. Calcium flows into the nerve terminal and leads to the release of a chemical called a *neurotransmitter*, which moves across the gap between the two nerves and binds to receptors in the postsynaptic membrane. This binding action works like the turning of a key in a lock, in that it has highly specific effect.

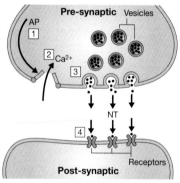

Fig. 4.3 Highly simplified diagram of a synapse (based on [1,43]). 1) An action potential AP arrives at the pre-synaptic membrane (Pre). 2) Calcium channels open. 3) Vesicles respond to the increased concentration of calcium by releasing neurotransmitters NT. 4) Neurotransmitters diffuse across the synaptic gap. They bind with receptors on the post-synaptic membrane (Post), leading to a reaction in the next nerve.

However, in the clinic this type of knowledge is of limited value, so the chapter includes models that can be more easily applied to the patient. The phenomenon of referred pain, so common in patients, is dealt with as well.

One cannot be certain about the processes taking place in a patient's spinal cord. However, there are signs and symptoms that enable the clinician to make an educated guess and these are discussed near the end of the chapter. Suggestions are made regarding the management of these findings.

EARLY INSIGHTS INTO SPINAL CORD FUNCTION

On a gross anatomical level, the dorsal horn can be seen as a relay station. It is the place where peripheral afferents enter the spinal cord, i.e. where signals are passed on to the central nervous system (Fig. 4.1). Most nociceptive fibres of type C and A delta synapse with a secondary neurone, which cross the midline and go up to the brain stem. Box 4.1 gives an overview of synaptic function. Information from mechanical receptors is passed on by A beta fibres that go directly to the dorsal column, not linking with secondary neurones until they reach the brain stem.

From an anatomical point of view, the dorsal horn seems to do little more than pass on the information that comes in from the periphery. The model of evolution described in previous chapters applies here as well. The phylogenetically older nociceptive fibres have to synapse and cross over before ascending. On the other hand, the more modern A beta fibres go straight to the brain, with a small collateral influencing the dorsal horn (Fig. 4.2).

Knowledge of spinal cord tracts and how they relate to sensation is based on the observations of the French surgeon Brown-Séquard

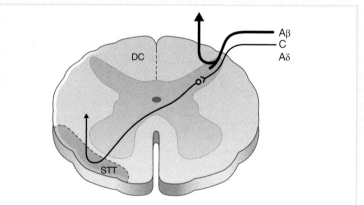

Fig. 4.1 Simplified cross section through the spinal cord. A beta fibres follow the dorsal column DC to the brain stem. Nociceptive fibres (C, A delta) links with a secondary neurone, which crosses the spinal cord diagonally and ascends in the spinothalamic tract STT.

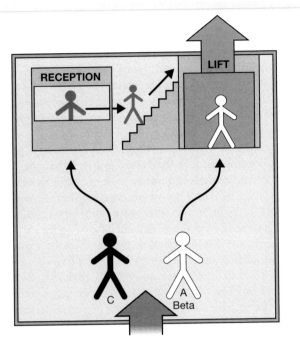

Fig. 4.2 Analogy explaining differences between two sensory pathways. The reception area of an office building representing the dorsal horn receives information from two sources. Couriers from company 'C' (nociceptive information) have to pass their messages to a receptionist, who has to run up the stairs to reach the manager (the brain). In contrast, couriers from 'A beta' (mechanoreceptor information) have a dedicated lift to the manager near the top. They inform the receptionist that they are going up (local collateral), but do not need her to pass the message on. The system used by C is the least efficient and used only in extreme circumstances.

(1817–1894). He tried to understand the signs and symptoms found in patients with partial spinal cord lesions, such as those resulting from bayonet or bullet wounds.[2,3] Apart from paralysis and vasomotor changes because of interrupted innervation, he would observe strange patterns of sensory change. A person with a transection of the left half of the spinal cord, would have an anaesthesized area on the same side, corresponding with the area innervated by the damaged nerve root. This was in line with what common sense would suggest. Fine touch would not be felt below that level on the same side, because the afferent information could not get past the lesion. What must have intrigued Brown-Séquard though, was the fact that on the side opposite to the lesion there was no sensitivity to temperature or pain, while the ability to feel light touch was unaffected. He concluded that the nerves for temperature and pain crossed the centre line at spinal cord level, before ascending to the brain stem (Fig. 4.1).

This type of anatomical knowledge dominated the field of neurology for a long time. It is of interest to the neurosurgeon, whose scalpel must carefully target specific structures and avoid others. The musculoskeletal clinician on the other hand, is more interested in assessing and influencing the *function* of this system. Indeed, although anatomical divisions clearly exist, they explain only a very small part of neural function in patients with pain.

The anatomical basis of pain perception was refined by the English neurologist Henry Head, who described the two components of pain discussed in Chapter 2.[4] He differentiated between short lasting, well localized epicritic pain transmitted by A delta fibres and slow onset, longer lasting and more diffuse protopathic pain from C fibre activation. It is interesting to note that Head warned that the division of protopathic and epicritic could not be maintained in the central nervous system. This was based on his observation that the separation of the two types of pain found after peripheral nerve lesions, as described in Chapter 3, was never present after a lesion of the central nervous system.[4,5] Head concluded that the two types of pain recombined once they entered the spinal cord. Here was an expert in neurology who concluded that anatomical divisions did not fully explain neural function.

For many years, the warnings against a rigid mechanistic view of the central nervous system did not have any great impact on the way pain was explained, even though it was clear that a number of pain related phenomena could not be explained. For example, for some patients the most innocuous stimuli such as brushing the skin could be painful. If the pain system was anatomically separate from the system dealing with normal sensation, how could this be explained?[6] Another issue was that the neuro-anatomical approach to treatment, consisting of division of peripheral nerves, sensory nerve root or even spinal cord, would often be unsuccessful in relieving pain.

Melzack and Wall attempted to think outside the confines of anatomical knowledge and developed a hypothetical model that was based on observations of function as well as physiology.[7] This model postulated interaction between small and large fibre input, as well as a regulating influence from the brain. It was called the Gate Control Theory of Pain. They incorporated the great variability in the relationship between stimulus and perceived pain in their model, in acknowledgement of the fact that in the world outside the laboratory an enormous variety could be observed.[8] In the extreme, injury may not be accompanied by pain and pain can exist in absence of injury. In addition, pain and tenderness associated with injury can spread in absence of changes to surrounding tissues, which suggests that innocuous mechanical stimuli could contribute to the perception of pain. On the other hand, stimulation of A beta innervated mechanoreceptors has the capacity to reduce pain as well, for instance when a painful area is rubbed.

Melzack and Wall faced fierce opposition from traditionalists, because their model flew in the face of the accepted neuro-anatomical idea of a hard-wired pain system. Although the Gate Control Theory explained some of the enigmas mentioned above, it was based on neural networks that were hypothetical and therefore difficult to defend. However, as science advanced it was discovered that although these networks did not exist in the exact form Melzack and Wall predicted, innocuous and nociceptive sensation did in fact combine in the dorsal horn. The dorsal horn turned out to be a centre of sensory integration and modification.[9] An interesting overview of the enormous amount of research that was inspired by the Gate Control Theory is provided by the Patrick Wall tribute issue of the journal *Pain*.[10]

Until the Gate Control Theory began to have an impact, the sensory nervous system was seen as a signalling structure that simply passed information from periphery to brain. Consequently, treatment of pain was based on suppression with drugs and the destruction of peripheral and central neural pathways. After the formulation of the Gate Control Theory, it became clear that the nervous system could actively modify pain. The understanding that certain stimuli could suppress pain at the level of the spinal cord led to greater understanding and acceptance of stimulation therapies such as acupuncture, electrotherapy and manual therapy. It also became clear that psychological interventions had a genuine effect on the way the nervous system processed pain.[11] The way that pain was regarded and treated had been changed forever.

DORSAL HORN SIGNALLING PATHWAYS

It is interesting that the specificity theory, based on the idea that pain and mechanosensitivity had their own separate pathways in the central nervous system, held sway for many years even though clinical observation contradicted it. When Melzack and Wall published a theory which demanded interaction between these two types of sensation, they put the spotlight on these contradictions. Both camps felt that they were representing the truth, yet their views seemed irreconcilable.

It could be said that reality encompasses both points of view. There is a degree of specificity in the central nervous system, yet the potential for interaction and overlapping is built in. It is a rich source of apparent paradoxes.

The classical idea of the dorsal horn as represented in Fig. 4.1 can be verified anatomically and seems to justify the original specificists' stance. However, with advancing physiological technology it has become possible to map the neurones in the dorsal horn more precisely. A slightly more detailed diagram shows that nociceptive information can in fact be passed on via two different secondary pathways (Fig. 4.4). *Nociceptive specific* (NS) nerves, which respond purely to nociceptive information from thin high threshold peripheral nerves, form the type of dedicated pain pathway represented in Fig. 4.1. On the other hand, many nociceptive fibres make contact with *Wide dynamic range* (WDR) nerve cells. Although they follow a pathway through the spinal cord similar to the NS cells, they are functionally very different.

Depolarization of the presynaptic nerve terminal triggers the release of a neurotransmitter, which binds with its specific type of receptor on the postsynaptic terminal. Many receptors are linked directly with an ion channel (see Ch. 2). The opening of a receptor channel creates a current which either increases or decreases the post-synaptic membrane potential.[12] Some neurotransmitters bind with receptors that reduce the membrane potential and make depolarization more likely. This is called an *Excitatory Post Synaptic Potential* or *EPSP*. The most common neurotransmitter that opens excitatory receptor channels in the dorsal horn is *glutamate*.

Other neurotransmitters such as *GABA* (*gamma-aminobutyric acid*) open channels that hyperpolarize the postsynaptic membrane potential, making depolarization less likely (*Inhibitory Post Synaptic Potential* or *IPSP*). Stimulation of a nerve that releases GABA therefore has a paradoxical effect. It reduces the chance that the postsynaptic cell depolarizes. In other words, stimulation of one nerve can lead to the reduced activity of another.

EPSPs are counteracted by IPSPs because their effects are 'added up' by the post-synaptic membrane. This summation affects potentials that arrive simultaneously. It is called *spatial summation* because it concerns addition of impulses simultaneously arriving at different locations. However, because it takes the membrane a short time to return to its resting state after a small change in potential, potentials that arrive in quick succession may also accumulate. This is known as *temporal summation* or addition over time. In the clinic, temporal summation may manifest as pain that increases with each repetition of a test. Some patients report little or no pain when tests are applied, but get increasingly uncomfortable as the examination progresses.

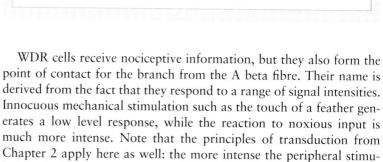

Fig. 4.4 A simplified model of sensory transmission at spinal cord level. Nociceptive fibres, represented as a single fibre C for clarity, can synapse with two types of secondary nerve, Nociceptive Specific (NS) and Wide Dynamic Range (WDR). NS cells receive only thin fibre input, while WDR cells also respond to A beta fibre stimulation via a collateral branch.

WDR cells receive nociceptive information, but they also form the point of contact for the branch from the A beta fibre. Their name is derived from the fact that they respond to a range of signal intensities. Innocuous mechanical stimulation such as the touch of a feather generates a low level response, while the reaction to noxious input is much more intense. Note that the principles of transduction from Chapter 2 apply here as well: the more intense the peripheral stimulation, the higher the impulse frequency in the nervous system.

Figure 4.4 makes it clear that those in favour of specificity are partially justified. Information from A beta fibres has its own pathway up to the thalamus, as do nociceptive signals. However, these two types of sensory input also share a pathway that starts with the WDR cell, which responds proportionately to the input it receives. This WDR cell is the place where the sensory interaction described in the Gate Theory takes place. The intriguing question is how this enables one person to control pain by 'rubbing it better', while some patients find that even light touch is painful. The interaction between nociceptive and innocuous sensation is not straightforward.

PAIN RELIEF FROM STIMULATION

The description of the dorsal horn given in the previous section makes it understandable how activity in primary afferents can generate action potentials in the WDR cells. Activity in one nerve creates activity in the next. What has not been made clear is how *stimulation* of A beta fibres can lead to a *reduction* in pain perception. This phenomenon relies on the presence of local nerves with an inhibitory influence. A second factor is the way the WDR cell functions, which will be discussed later in this chapter.

Figure 4.4. shows the A beta fibre connecting directly with the WDR cell. In reality, many A beta fibres have additional synapses with *inhibitory interneurones*. These nerves form short links between the primary and secondary nerve, or between an A beta neurone and a

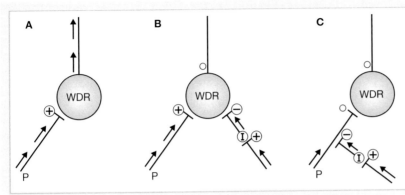

Fig. 4.5 Inhibitory interneurones (based on [44]). **A.** Stimulation of primary neurone P depolarizes the secondary nerve WDR. **B.** Post-synaptic inhibition. Simultaneous stimulation of an inhibitory interneurone I counteracts depolarization in the WDR cell. **C.** Pre-synaptic inhibition. Stimulation of an inhibitory interneurone prevents the action potential in P from reaching the WDR cell.

nociceptive nerve (Fig. 4.5). While primary neurones (C, A delta and A beta) release neurotransmitters that lower the stimulation threshold in the nerve, they synapse with and facilitate depolarization, the neurotransmitters by inhibitory interneurones have the opposite effect (Box 4.2).

The WDR cell combines the inputs from many primary neurones and interneurones. In effect, it is a small decision making centre because it 'weighs up' the balance of the incoming information. Many nerves synapse with the WDR cell. Input from a single neurone has little effect, unless this input is supported by input from several others. One could say that the information is passed on, only if it is 'sanctioned' by other sources. On the other hand, if the information is not supported, or even countered by inhibitory impulses, it may get blocked. Figure 4.6 shows the potential complexity involved in the integration of many nerve impulses.

The pain relieving effect of selective A beta fibre stimulation can be explained by the fact that these nerves activate inhibitory interneurones, which in turn reduce the membrane potential of the WDR. This is thought to be an important mechanism underlying the pain relieving effect of massage and other manual interventions. The understanding of the neurophysiological effect of mechanical therapies has

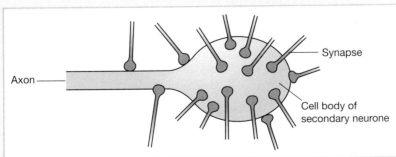

Axon

Synapse

Cell body of secondary neurone

Fig. 4.6 Many neurones influence a single secondary nerve cell (based on figure on p. 651 in [45]).

led to their re-evaluation as *stimulation therapies*, rather than just mechanical therapies. This has increased their acceptance by the medical profession. It is therefore even more regrettable that many of the physical therapists themselves persist in using strictly mechanical paradigms. Other forms of stimulation therapy are Transcutaneous Electrical Nerve Stimulation (TENS), and acupuncture.

Unfortunately, stimulation-induced inhibition of the WDR as outlined here can only explain the pain relieving effect of mechanical treatments *while they are being applied*. After all, A beta activity drops down to normal level as soon as the treatment is over. Therefore, this inhibitory mechanism does not explain the long-term effects of the physical therapies on pain (for an interesting discussion on this topic, see [13]). These effects are more likely to be mediated by activation of certain brain structures, which play an important role in the control of pain. Chapter 8 discusses cerebral brain control in some detail.

ALLODYNIA: PAIN FROM INNOCUOUS STIMULATION

Interestingly, while some patients get relief from stimulation therapies, others experience quite the opposite. For those people, even the most innocent of stimuli can cause pain. Damage to a peripheral nerve is one of the possible causes of this phenomenon called allodynia, as discussed in the previous chapter. Another potential mechanism is a change in dorsal horn function. Just as A beta stimulation can influence the way nociceptive information is processed, is nociception capable of changing how A beta information is dealt with.

When both nociceptive and A beta stimulation arrive at the same WDR cell, the outcome depends on the balance of stimuli. If the inhibitory influence from the A beta fibres and the inhibitory interneurones prevails, the WDR's response is subdued. This influence does not only rely on the input from the periphery, but is also determined by controlling nerves from the brain. The discussion in this chapter focuses on segmental processes and inhibition by the brain will be dealt with in Chapter 8.

The balance may also tip towards the noxious stimulation. If the WDR membrane potential is lowered considerably because of strong and persistent input from nociceptive fibres, the A beta input may lower it even further. Two mechanisms have been identified as potentially involved in the development of this so-called *central sensitization*. One is called *wind up*, the other *long-term potentiation (LTP)*.

Wind up is a phenomenon that has been observed in laboratory settings. When a C fibre is stimulated repeatedly at a relatively high frequency, it continues to depolarize even when stimulation has ceased. This spontaneous firing can take a long time to fizzle out and it can be maintained by successive stimulation. In other words, although it takes intense and high frequency stimulation for a C fibre to go into a state of wind up, it requires much less to maintain. An analogy would be getting a heavy flywheel or a car to move by pushing it (the reader should try this if in doubt, remembering to take off the brakes first). Initially it takes a lot of effort to get going, but once it moves relatively little effort is required.

It is interesting to note that wind up develops whether a person is conscious or not. A person undergoing surgery may develop long lasting sensitization of the dorsal horns supplying the operation site with sensory nerves, *even though they are under general anaesthetic.* In

The main neurotransmitter released by C fibres that has an excitatory effect is called glutamate. It binds to receptors on ion channels in the membrane of the secondary neurone. There are two types of ion channel, AMPA (alpha-amino-3-hydroxy-5-methylisoxazole-4-propionic acid) and NMDA (N-methyl-D-aspartate).[12] Under normal circumstances, glutamate opens only the AMPA channels, because the NMDA channels are blocked by a magnesium molecule. A low membrane potential can remove this molecule, but usually the membrane returns to its resting state before this has happened.

Repeated stimulation in laboratory circumstances leads to temporal summation of EPSPs and lowers the membrane potential for longer than usual. This may give the NMDA channels enough time to expel their magnesium molecule. Once more channels are unblocked, the release of a small amount of glutamate by the primary nerve leads to a much greater response in the secondary nerve (Fig. 4.7).

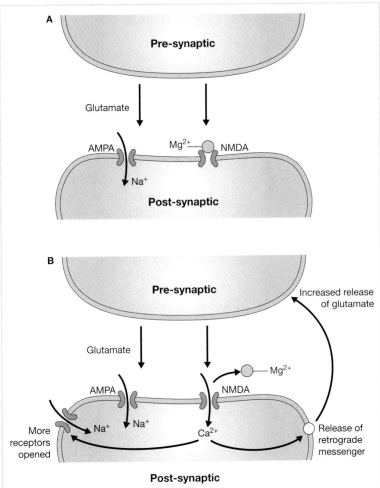

Fig. 4.7 The role of NMDA channels. **A.** Nociceptive stimulation leads to the release of glutamate, which opens AMPA channels. The NMDA channels remain blocked by magnesium (Mg^{2+}). **B.** Persistent stimulation causes the ejection of magnesium, creating an influx of calcium (Ca^{2+}). As long as the channels remain unblocked, a small amount of glutamate has a greater effect than when only the AMPA channels are opened. Increased levels of intracellular calcium trigger processes inside the post-synaptic cell, leading to a greater response. They also trigger the release of retrograde messengers that facilitate the release of glutamate from the pre-synaptic membrane.

an effort to reduce the incidence of persistent post-surgical pain, the use of pre-emptive analgesia is now advocated by the International Association for the Study of Pain.[14]

LTP is thought to be the result of wind up and other forms of persistent nociceptive stimulation. The bombardment of the secondary neurone with glutamate opens more ion channels in its membrane than when stimulation is of shorter duration and lower intensity (Box 4.3). The result is an ever increasing calcium influx into the secondary cell, which makes it even more excitable.[15,16] Eventually this hyperexcitable state is thought to lead to the release of a so-called retrograde messenger, which diffuses back to the primary nerve, causing it to release more neurotransmitter when an impulse arrives. This closes a self-perpetuating feedback loop of sensitization. At a later stage, the connection may be strengthened even further by the formation of new synapses.[17]

THE DORSAL HORN AS AMPLIFIER: STATE DEPENDENT PROCESSING

The molecular mechanisms described above can seem far removed from the realities of clinical practice. Physical therapists are not in a position to prescribe drugs that target these mechanisms. Establishing whether they play a role is not possible with any amount of certainty. Nevertheless, an understanding of dorsal horn changes can lead the therapist away from tissue-focused thinking and closer to mechanism based approaches. The explanation of central mechanisms to the patient can also have a powerful effect on the impact of the pain.[18,19]

The development of simplified models makes the integration of knowledge about central changes into clinical reasoning and patient explanation much easier. One such model is the concept of the dorsal horn as an amplifier of incoming information, as discussed in this section. The section, The dorsal horn as selector, below deals with an equally useful model of changing selectivity.

Under normal circumstances, sensory input is processed in the dorsal horn as expected from a classical point of view. Mechanical stimuli of low intensity affect A beta fibres and lead to normal sensation. For example, touch is perceived as touch and stretch as stretch. The intensity of the stimulus corresponds with the intensity of the felt sensation. When the stimulation becomes extremely intense or is damaging, it activates a dedicated nociceptive system of C and A delta fibres and causes pain.

The fact that this clear linear correspondence between stimulus and felt sensation exists in most people most of the time, creates the illusion of a hardwired nervous system. A more realistic view is that sensations are processed in a variable way, rather than according to immutable principles. In the dorsal horn, the nervous system makes an *active decision* about the way incoming information is processed. The normal correspondence between stimulus and sensation is therefore not an absolute given, but exists only because the dorsal horn makes it happen.

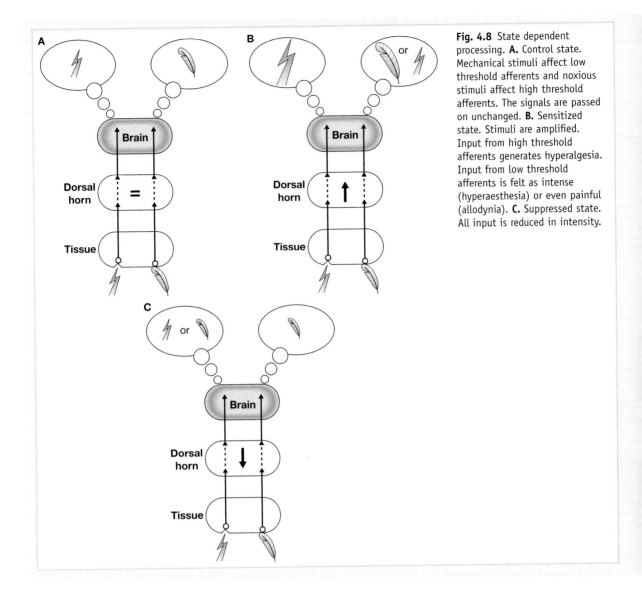

Fig. 4.8 State dependent processing. **A.** Control state. Mechanical stimuli affect low threshold afferents and noxious stimuli affect high threshold afferents. The signals are passed on unchanged. **B.** Sensitized state. Stimuli are amplified. Input from high threshold afferents generates hyperalgesia. Input from low threshold afferents is felt as intense (hyperaesthesia) or even painful (allodynia). **C.** Suppressed state. All input is reduced in intensity.

One of the ways in which the dorsal horn can influence sensation, is by changing the amplification of the incoming signals. This is similar to turning the volume control of a sound system up or down. Clifford Woolf has called this *state dependent processing*.[16,20] He describes four processing states (Fig. 4.8).

Normal processing takes place when the dorsal horn is in its *physiological state* or *control state*. However, under certain circumstances the dorsal horn may amplify incoming impulses. In this *sensitized state*, a stimulus will feel stronger than it actually is. This is sometimes called *central sensitization*, the increased sensitivity of the central nervous system.

This sensitized state can be observed in some patients with persistent pain. Normal stimuli are perceived as disproportionately strong, a

Table 4.1 Types of sensation mediated by A beta fibres (after [50,51])

Skin and subcutaneous tissues	Muscle, joint
Stroking	Stretch, angle
Pressure	Movement
Vibration	Capsule stretch
Stretch	

Box 4.4 Synaptic correlates of learning

It may seem counterintuitive that persistent painful input leads to sensitization and therefore to more easily felt pain. However, LTP is the same process underlying learning.[17] When a person tries to learn a task, certain groups of synapses are activated repeatedly. After a while, the synapses involved become sensitized and can be activated by a low level of stimulation. For example, the amount of deliberate control required to learn to play a musical instrument is enormous compared with that of the experienced musician. If the new activity continues to be used the process is facilitated by the formation of more synapses, thereby hard-wiring the networks and therefore the required skills.

The same mechanisms are involved when certain neural pathways are repeatedly activated by nociceptive input. Central sensitization therefore is a process of adaptation, just like learning. From the point of view of evolution and survival, it makes sense to be able to respond more easily to a nociceptive stimulus that is experienced regularly. This learning process does not only take place in the brain, but also in other parts of the central nervous system, such as the dorsal horn.

phenomenon known as hyperaesthesia. The stimulation of A beta fibres, which normally transmit innocuous mechanical information, may create a stronger sensation than normally expected. It may even be amplified to such a degree that it is perceived as painful, which is known as mechanical allodynia. At the same time, the input from nociceptive neurones into the dorsal horn may also be amplified, which makes painful stimuli feel even more painful, a phenomenon known as *secondary hyperalgesia*. This type of increased pain response is different from primary hyperalgesia, which is the result of sensitization of the peripheral nerve endings (see Ch. 2).

It is common for clinicians to assume that hyperaesthesia, hyperalgesia and allodynia relate to touch, i.e. to the skin. However, Table 4.1 makes it clear that muscle spindles and joint capsules are also innervated by A beta fibres. These fibres follow a similar course to those from the skin. The implication for physical therapy is that stretching a muscle or joint capsule may cause pain when the dorsal horn innervating that structure is in a sensitized state. This pain can be generated in absence of any abnormality of the muscle or joint, or their innervating peripheral nerves. In other words, a sensitized dorsal horn can easily lead to *false positives* in the objective examination. Fortunately, knowledge of the manifestations of sensitization discussed later in this chapter and careful clinical reasoning enable the clinician to generate appropriate clinical hypotheses and strategies.

State dependent processing has equally important consequences for treatment. If the main factor maintaining pain and sensitivity is not tissue pathology but rather the processing state of the dorsal horn, treatment of the tissues is misguided. Instead, the aim of the treatment should be to bring the dorsal horn back to its control state and restore normal sensory function. Even when genuine tissue pathology exists in addition to sensitization, dorsal horn function has to be addressed. After all, sensitization can negate the pain relieving effects of mechanical and anti-inflammatory treatments. It may not respond to treatments of the tissues.

The dorsal horn also has the ability to attenuate incoming signals. When it enters a *suppressed state*, the stimulation of low threshold afferents results in a faint sensation. This is called hypoaesthesia. Nociceptive signals may be similarly reduced, in which case it is referred to as hypoalgesia, i.e. pain feels less strong than it normally would. The dorsal horn may even suppress information to such an extent that it is not perceived at all.

The fourth state described by Woolf is called *remodelling*. This is similar to the sensitized state, with an important difference. When pain persists, the dorsal horn may grow new nerves and connections.[16,21] In addition, persistent release of glutamate leads to so-called *excitotoxicity*, toxic levels of excitatory neurotransmitter.[22] This may cause the destruction of inhibitory neurones in the dorsal horn, which effectively robs the central nervous system of its pain controlling mechanism.[23] While sensitization is a functional change that can be reversed at any time, remodelling is thought to make the amplification more permanent and potentially hard to treat. In the analogy of the sound system, sensitization corresponds with turning up the volume. Remodelling is similar to changing the amplifier internally, so that a minimum volume is produced even when you turn the control right down. Effective pain control can prevent these changes, but it is not certain whether it can reverse them.

It may seem strange that the nervous system creates a situation where pain is felt more easily. In fact, sensitization and remodelling are forms of functional adaptation to potentially important information that is received frequently or persistently, similar to a learning process (Box 4.4). If a person perceives or does something frequently, recognition of the stimulus and responses become easier. After a while, it may even become automatic. This is the result of synaptic changes, which make it increasingly easy for the relevant signals to be passed on. This also applies when these relevant signals are nociceptive information: the nervous system learns to facilitate the processing of pain. As a result, a patient may feel pain at the slightest of touches, or when put in circumstances very similar to the ones that created the pain in the first instance.

Viewing pain as the result of a learning process has implications for the way treatments are conceptualized. Effective treatment of the tissues can be seen as taking away the conditioning stimulus that feeds this learning. Another approach to treatment involves reducing the importance of the stimulus, which takes away the need for constant attention. Examples of this method are explanation, psychological intervention and distraction.

THE DORSAL HORN AS SELECTOR

Enhanced sensory processing in the dorsal horn does not limit itself to amplification of the afferent input, but may also involve a reduction in selectivity (Box 4.5). This means that the dorsal horn has difficulty keeping separate the multitude of signals that it receives.

Sensitization of the dorsal horn is associated with a reduction in its selectivity. Irwin Korr referred to this as the 'facilitated segment'.[24] Signals that were previously filtered out are now passed on. Allodynia may be interpreted as a reduction in selectivity. For example, one can

Box 4.5 Selectivity

To understand the concept of selectivity, it may be helpful to think of trying to tune in to a radio station. A highly selective radio receiver will be able to pick up one station, even if another station is very close to it on the dial. On the other hand, a radio of poorer quality may not be as selective and either produce the sound of both stations simultaneously or continually switch between the two.

In the control state, the dorsal horn is highly selective. High numbers of sensory neurones from a variety of tissues enter a very small area of spinal cord. Some information is filtered out, because it is not important. For example, the sensation of the clothes one is wearing, the constant ticking of a clock in the room and the actions of one's bowels don't normally require attention. Sensations from myotomes, sclerotomes and dermatomes are kept separate and the person is able to distinguish between them.

Box 4.6 Referred pain

Referred pain can be defined as the perception of pain at a distance from the location where the painful stimulus originates. It can either radiate from the pain site, or be perceived at some distance from it. The phenomenon is not purely subjective, because measurable referred tenderness and hyperalgesia may also be present.[25,26]

Pain refers from deep structures to ones that are more superficial:[27]

- Cutaneous pain does not refer.
- Muscle pain can be felt locally, but can also refer to other muscle regions and to a cutaneous area.
- Pain from visceral tissue is more likely to be felt in areas of referral than at the point of origin. It is often diffuse and poorly localized, because the viscera have few afferents and commonly share sensory pathways with somatic structures.[28,29] Pain can refer to muscles and skin.

It is thought that convergence of innervation from different types of tissue onto a limited number of dorsal horn cells is responsible for the referral of pain. Pain is therefore most likely to be referred to segmentally related tissues. For example, the stomach has a thoracic innervation and can refer pain to the thoracic spine.[30] However, if the peritoneum, which is innervated by the phrenic nerve, is irritated as well, the pain may also refer to muscles and skin innervated by C2, 3 and 4.[31] The resulting clinical presentation may be confusing for the clinician. While treatment of the individual painful structures is frustrating, addressing the dorsal horn mechanisms at the centre of the plethora of problems may be more rewarding.

There are several conceptual models of referred pain, none of which explain all observed phenomena (Fig. 4.9).[30] The exact mechanism is still not known. The following overview is based on references [27,29]. The convergence-projection theory is based on the idea that somatic and visceral afferent information converges onto common secondary neurones, as found in several experimental studies.[32] The brain interprets pain from deep tissues such as muscles and viscera as stemming from structures that are more superficial. This theory is plausible, but does not explain the development of measurable hyperalgesia in the referral area.

A slightly different model that is able to account for referred hyperalgesia, is the convergence-facilitation theory. It suggests that nociceptive input from viscera may cause central sensitization, which causes normal somatic input to be perceived as painful.

A related model, the thalamic convergence theory, ascribes referred sensation to summation of inputs in the thalamus rather than in the spinal cord. This theory explains several characteristics of referred pain, but it fails to account for the reduction in referred pain intensity after the application of local anaesthetics or a tourniquet.[33]

The axon reflex theory is based on the assumption that some afferent nerves are bifurcated, innervating both visceral and somatic tissues. Although this type of axon does exist, its prevalence is extremely limited.

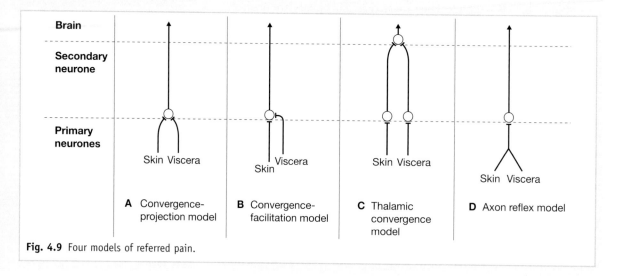

Fig. 4.9 Four models of referred pain.

become more aware of clothes touching the skin. This touch can even become an annoyance. Similarly, signals from deep inside the body that were previously suppressed may make themselves felt. Reduced selectivity means that the nervous system is no longer able to separate these inputs and signals from viscera, muscles and skin begin to influence each other where they enter the spinal cord. This results in so-called *referred pain* and *referred tenderness* (Box 4.6).

Patients may give a hint that their selectivity is low by saying that they cannot tell where the pain is coming from. The pain seems to come from a diffuse region rather than a well-defined location. The clinician is likely to find a generalized tenderness or soreness and elicit pain from a variety of tests. What these positive tests may have in common is their spinal innervation levels, rather than a mechanical interaction. Treatment can be conceptualized as bringing the selectivity back to normal, either by normalizing sensory input or by reducing the perceived need to focus on all incoming information.

SYMPTOMS SUGGESTIVE OF CENTRAL INVOLVEMENT

Traditionally, the medical profession has taken a 'them or us' approach to pain. No pain is good, while pain is generally considered bad and associated with injury and disease. If nothing can be done about the pathology, then at least the pain should be fought and suppressed. Given that the nervous system may naturally make active changes to enhance or generate pain, this 'war on pain' is also a war on normal sensory function. It is questionable whether this is the correct way to deal with the body.

As demonstrated in this and the previous chapter, the nervous system actively changes in response to events in the periphery. It has ways of increasing its sensitivity, if the sensory input is likely to be important. The implication is that the application of analgesics and pain suppressing modalities may go against the adaptation in the nervous system. In fact, the harder a physician works to suppress pain, the more the nervous system will try to extract information from the periphery by increasing its sensitivity. Ultimately, this results in increasing levels and areas of hyperaesthesia and hyperalgesia. Once the neural changes become structural, the pain may spiral out of control altogether.

It is therefore important to find out whether pain has a central component. If the nervous system is making efforts to reduce its selectivity and amplify incoming information, then simply treating the pain is likely to make matters worse. Instead, the dorsal horn must be enticed to settle down and return to focused and controlled function. The identification of sensitization is the subject of this section, while the next section makes suggestions for treatment.

Certain descriptions in the patient's history are suggestive of a central element in the maintenance of pain. If present, these 'central flags' may be followed up in the examination of the patient.

- Pain may start as a soft tissue injury, inflammation or damage to a nerve. If pain persists beyond the expected healing time, processing changes in the dorsal horn may maintain it. As discussed in the previous chapters, inflammation and neuropathy are in themselves associated with sensory changes. Although it is not possible to separate central and peripheral contributions to a patient's pain with certainty in a clinical situation, a clear understanding of the characteristics of nociceptive and peripheral neurogenic pain should enable an educated guess.

- Central changes occur not only in response to peripheral, but also to central events. The brain exerts facilitatory and inhibitory influences on the dorsal horn via descending nerves (see Ch. 8). A person's state of mind, previous experiences and expectation are capable of altering sensory transmission at the level of the spinal cord. It can be helpful to place oneself in the position of the patient, asking whether suppression of pain is likely. For example, the nervous system of a patient who is concerned that they have a spinal fracture is most likely to facilitate and amplify any sensation coming from the back. For such a patient, only effective, patient-focused reassurance can start a normalization of dorsal horn function.

- Patients may find it difficult to tell where their pain is coming from: the pain seems to come from a diffuse region rather than a well-defined location. Although it is recommended that the patient be asked whether the main pain can be identified by pointing with one finger, it is a mistake to insist on precision if the patient indicates a vague pain distribution.

- Sometimes patients struggle to find words to describe their pain, because central changes alter pain perception. The quality and behaviour of the symptoms associated with central changes may not be like somatic sensations, even though the brain places them in the body's tissues. As discussed in the previous chapter, difficulty in matching a sensation with a description does not indicate lack of intelligence or education, but must be interpreted as a positive indicator that the patient experiences a sensation or sensations that they are utterly unfamiliar with.

- Pain may spread to segmentally related structures, but also to adjoining spinal levels. Each peripheral nerve enters the spine at up to five levels, so each point on the body is innervated by a maximum of five segments.[34] Segments are also linked by so-called *propriospinal nerves* within the spinal cord. It is likely that loss of selectivity involves a disinhibition of these intersegmental links, resulting in a more generalized response to sensory impulses. An example is the person described in Box 3.5 who has widespread pains following a small incision.

- Sensory input from the same segment and eventually neighbouring segments may contribute to the pain. Initially, a patient with an injured ankle ligament is likely to feel pain when the ankle is moved. If the pain persists, stimulation of segmentally related structures, i.e. muscles innervated by the same spinal nerve, can aggravate it. Eventually, stimulation of tissues innervated by adjoining segments may also begin to contribute, so that the stretch or contraction of other muscles or the stretch of other ankle ligaments becomes painful. This is not a purely subjective finding; the uninjured structures can become hyperaesthetic.

- The patient is likely to describe a lack of response to analgesics. Normal analgesics and anti-inflammatory drugs are thought to act mainly in the periphery. Therefore, if a patient benefits from these types of drug, central changes are unlikely to play a major role in the maintenance of their pain.
- The patient may have a history of failed manual treatments. Local mechanical treatments may or may not be of help for centrally maintained pain, depending on its target and a variety of factors beyond the therapist's control. A treatment focused purely on the release of soft tissues including the mechanical interfaces of peripheral nerves, may or may not alter the pain. If the dorsal horn is in a sensitized state, intensive physical therapy is likely to represent an increased sensory barrage that maintains or increases pain. It is possible that response to treatment is erratic, in that a treatment may seem effective for a limited period, but not when it is repeated.
- In musculoskeletal structures, facilitation by the dorsal horn may manifest in the form of active *myofascial trigger points*, which have

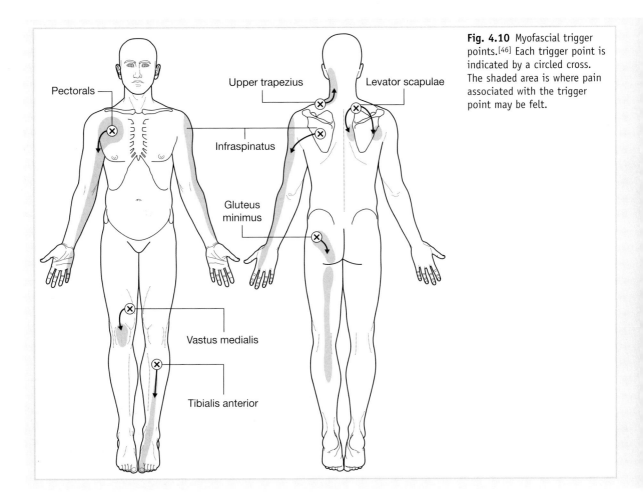

Fig. 4.10 Myofascial trigger points.[46] Each trigger point is indicated by a circled cross. The shaded area is where pain associated with the trigger point may be felt.

Pectorals

Upper trapezius

Levator scapulae

Infraspinatus

Gluteus minimus

Vastus medialis

Tibialis anterior

a characteristic pattern of referral (Fig. 4.10). Active trigger points can be characterized as follows:[35]

Trigger points may develop in any soft tissue including periosteum. The point is exquisitely tender and may elicit a flinch on palpation. There is pain in a characteristic distribution around or distant from the point.
Pain referral may be reproduced by mechanical irritation of the point, such as palpation.
Muscles often develop a palpable taut band around the trigger point and become generally shortened.

- Referred pain and tenderness may be the result of visceral pathology. Maps of visceral referred pain were first developed by Henry Head in the late 19th century (Fig. 4.11). He compared regions of cutaneous hyperalgesia in patients with visceral pathology with the distribution of herpes zoster lesions in other patients.[30] If a patient's symptoms do not follow a consistent musculoskeletal pattern, careful questioning may bring to light a visceral problem. Further advice is given in Chapter 5.

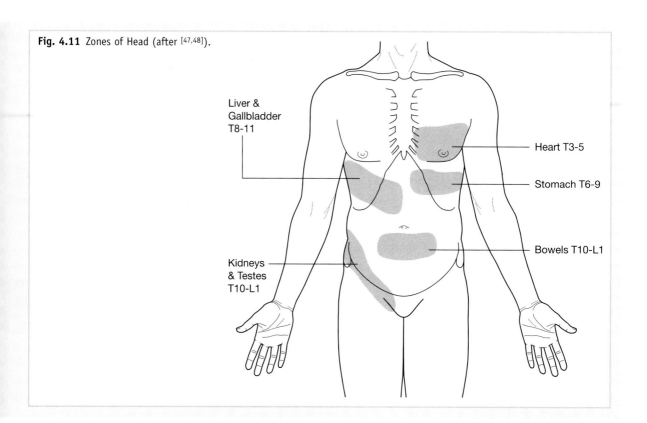

Fig. 4.11 Zones of Head (after [47,48]).

Liver & Gallbladder T8-11

Heart T3-5

Stomach T6-9

Bowels T10-L1

Kidneys & Testes T10-L1

EXAMINATION

Careful history taking, complemented by a thorough physical examination and sound clinical reasoning, should enable the clinician to
establish whether the patient's symptoms can be *fully* explained by
injury, inflammation and neuropathy. If the features do not fit completely, changes in central sensory processing have to be considered.

- The time course of the pain may not be directly related to an individual stimulus applied to somatic structures. The phenomena of temporal summation and wind up explains why pain may persist for
  longer than expected, for instance after palpation or the application
  of manual tests. Some patients experience this as an 'echo' of the pain
  or afterpain. Therapists are advised to be gentle with patients suspected of dorsal horn changes, because the impact of a technique on
  the pain may not be apparent until after its application.
- Sensitivity may be found in structures and organs that are linked by
  their segmental innervation. It is therefore important that clinicians
  know innervation levels of musculoskeletal and cutaneous regions.
- Musculoskeletal trigger points create a predictable pattern of pain referral, which can be either provoked or spontaneous (see above). Careful
  palpation can identify trigger points and elicit referred pain. Care must
  be taken to distinguish this from pain generated by the peripheral nerve
  by comparing the pattern of pain referral with peripheral innervation
  areas. Further sensory testing as suggested in Chapter 3 may be needed
  to eliminate doubt regarding the exact nature of the pain.

TREATMENT APPROACHES

Most of this chapter has concentrated on pain enhancing changes in
the dorsal horn. However, there are influences that enable the central
nervous system to keep pain under control by turning down the amplification and narrowing the recruitment of inputs. These inhibitory
influences are of therapeutic value. They can be divided into two
categories: segmental and descending.

Segmental inhibition of pain was conceptualized by Melzack and
Wall[9]. Selective stimulation of myelinated fibres can inhibit the transmission of nociceptive information, when it enters the dorsal horn
at the same spinal level. This applies most clearly to A beta fibres,
which innervate mechanoreceptors. However, A delta fibres share
some characteristics with A beta fibres at dorsal horn level and can
also provide inhibitory input.

Segmental inhibition means that the sensitivity of the dorsal horn
can be reduced by stimulation. Therefore, in order to understand the
influence that physical therapies can have on pain transmission, they
have to be viewed not just as mechanical treatments, but also as stimulation therapies. Another term for therapies that treat one part of the
body in order to achieve an effect elsewhere, is *reflex therapies*. An
example is acupuncture, in which needles stimulate certain nerves,
which in turn affect their innervation area and segmentally related

A patient presented in clinic with persistent and increasing anteromedial knee pain. The pain started after a knee arthroscopy. The therapist found it difficult to perform tests of the knee joint because most movements were painful, as was light touch of the painful area. He tried to give the patient some light knee exercises, but they caused too much pain.

The therapist decided to maximize A beta input into the affected spinal segments. He knew that the affected area was innervated by branches of the femoral nerve, which originates from L2, 3 and 4. He also realized that several adductor muscles, the iliopsoas and the tibialis anterior were innervated from these levels. He prescribed stretching exercises of the adductors and the iliopsoas, in a way that did not mechanically affect the knee joint. He also taught the patient how to use acupressure on points in the tibialis anterior muscle (Stomach 36, 37 and 38) and advised him to massage the non-painful areas of the thigh.

Once the patient established a routine, some simple stretches of the lumbar spine were added for further A beta input into the relevant spinal levels. Finally, applying the overflow principle used in neurological rehabilitation, the therapist gave the patient exercises to improve strength and balance of the unaffected leg.

After a few weeks, the pain and soreness had settled sufficiently to allow further examination of the knee and start some more localized treatment.

structures.[36] Electrical stimulation such as TENS can be applied in a similar way.

Manual techniques can be interpreted as nerve stimulation in the same way as electrotherapy or acupuncture. A beta innervated mechanoreceptors are stimulated by pressure, stretch and stroking of the skin, all of which are used in manual therapy. Similarly, movement and moderate stretch of muscle, joint capsule and ligament are forms of A beta fibre stimulation. Once the innervation level of the painful or injured structure is known, manual treatments can be applied to other structures with the same segmental innervation. This creates A beta input into the segment, which inhibit the transmission of nociceptive information (Box 4.7).

Segmental treatment uses myotomes, dermatomes and 'arthrotomes' to affect sensory processing in the dorsal horn. Contralateral exercises may be added because the two sides of the spinal cord influence each other. The principle of treatment can be summarized as maximizing normal sensory input into the affected spinal levels. This input can be provided by applying manual techniques or electrical stimulation, but also by teaching the patient how to find and maintain good posture and movement without excessive compensation. Compensatory movements and positions are a form of abnormal input for the nervous system, stimulating muscle spindles and other mechanoreceptors in unusual patterns.

Segmental treatment need not limit itself to the stimulation of A beta fibres. A delta fibres are nociceptive, but also transmit high intensity non-noxious information. In the dorsal horn, they terminate in the same area as C fibres, but also where A beta fibres project. As a result, their function has both nociceptive and mechanoreceptor properties. It can be reasonably hypothesized that some high intensity treatment, creating what some patients call a 'nice pain' or 'healing pain', stimulate these fibres and have a powerful effect on the dorsal horn. An example is the Pressure Release Phenomenon described by Mulligan[37] and the release of trigger points with either pressure or acupuncture.[35]

As mentioned in the previous section, Henry Head developed maps of visceral referred pain. Max Kibler described in 1949 how warmth, massage and local anaesthetics could be applied to these so-called 'zones of Head' in order to treat the organ dysfunction that caused them.[38] In other words, Head's discovery concerned how the viscera influenced somatic sensation, while Kibler reversed the principle by using somatic stimulation to influence the viscera. This principle was developed fully in Connective Tissue Manipulation (CTM, Bindegewebsmassage) by Elizabeth Dicke and Hede Teirich-Leube.[38,39] CTM treatment stimulates the sensory nerves innervating cutaneous and fascial regions in order to have an effect on segmentally related organs and blood vessels. These so-called *connective tissue zones* correspond to a large extent with the zones described by Head.[40]

Myofascial release shares techniques with CTM, suggesting that its alleged effect on visceral function may be established via a neural

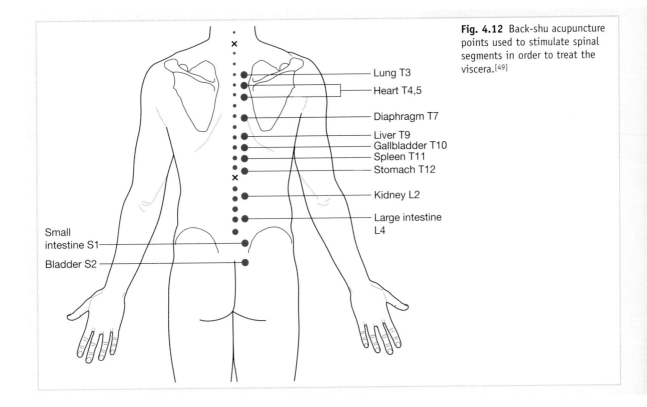

Fig. 4.12 Back-shu acupuncture points used to stimulate spinal segments in order to treat the viscera.[49]

Lung T3
Heart T4,5
Diaphragm T7
Liver T9
Gallbladder T10
Spleen T11
Stomach T12
Kidney L2
Large intestine L4
Small intestine S1
Bladder S2

rather than a mechanical route. Similarly, acupuncture points may be selected for the treatment of visceral problems on the basis of their segmental influence. The so-called *back-shu points* are all located along the spine. Each point and therefore each spinal level is described as influencing a particular internal organ. From a western perspective, each point creates an input into the main spinal segment innervating its viscera (Fig. 4.12).[36,41]

Whether an uncomfortable treatment succeeds in reducing pain, or whether it indeed aggravates it, depends on the balance of inputs into the dorsal horn. Segmental input is one form of input and descending inhibition is the other. The latter enables the brain to regulate its own input and control pain. This mechanism will be discussed in detail in Chapter 8. It may be activated in different circumstances and for different reasons.

One form of descending inhibition is known as stress-induced analgesia. This mechanism is activated in life threatening situations. Although it is effective, its application in acceptable forms of physical therapy is limited.

The brain may also suppress pain once the nature of the pain is clear, the level of concern is reduced and the person regains control. It is therefore important that therapists make every effort to explain their patient's symptoms and take away unhelpful fears and anxieties.

CONCLUSION

Persistent pain can cause changes in the dorsal horn that amplify and maintain the pain. Nerves that are not directly involved in the area generating the nociceptive stimulation become involved, leading to allodynia and hyperalgesia that spread outside their expected boundaries and an increasing gamut of influences on the pain. Forunately, segmental and descending inhibitory influences can keep these changes under control. Segmental stimulation is a part of any manual treatment, exercise routine or nerve stimulation, which may explain the beneficial effect these approaches can have on pain. However, their effect may be made explicit and maximized by interpreting musculoskeletal treatments as forms of reflex therapies. In addition, cognitive strategies can be utilized to activate descending inhibition.

The patient also needs active strategies, which can consist of mental and physical routines as well as work, leisure activities and education.

The chapters on psychology and the brain clarify these topics. For now, it is important that the therapist understands that these cerebral factors influence the way pain is processed in the dorsal horn. If a sensation such as pain is not of particular concern to the person or the organism, that sensation can be minimized by the nervous system. However, alarm and uncertainty puts that sensation under a magnifying glass by increasing amplification, and widens the influence of the pain by reducing selectivity.

In laboratory situations, dorsal horn changes can be produced by ongoing inflammation or neuropathy. Treatment of persistent pain is therefore often multifactorial. It may involve producing selective sensory stimulation in order to manipulate the activity in the dorsal horn, central inhibition by giving the patient more control through explanation, advice and exercises, and the reduction of nociceptive input by treating tissues and nerves.

Although normal analgesics are unlikely to have a lasting effect on centrally maintained pain, adjuvant medication such as tricyclic antidepressants and anticonvulsants mentioned in the previous chapter may be effective. This can be discussed with the patient's GP or specialist.

If a patient's pain has a central component, it is important that the patient is given an explanation of the mechanisms involved. State dependent processing and selectivity of the dorsal horn are models that can easily be translated so that the patient understands. Wind up is a model for pain that flares up after rather than during activity. It can be used to explain why overactivity on a 'good day' may lead to pain increases the day after.

Some therapists do not explain pain mechanisms to their patients, because they feel that they lack the intelligence or education required for understanding. This is an assumption that is unhelpful and often unjustified.[42] It is important that concerns and uncertainties are addressed in a way that connects with the individual. Even a person of low intelligence has a brain that modifies sensory input according to perceived need. In fact, such a person may find it more difficult to rationalize fears and need more rather than less cognitive input.

References

[1] Kandel E, Siegelbaum S. Overview of synaptic transmission. In: Kandel E, Schwartz J, Jessell T, eds. Principles of neural science. New York: McGraw-Hill 2000: 175–188

[2] Tattersall R, Turner B. Brown-Séquard and his syndrome. Lancet 2000; 356 (9223):61–63

[3] Head H, Thompson T. The interrelation of afferent impulses in their passage up the spinal cord. In: Head H, ed. Studies in neurology. London: Frowde/Hodder and Stoughton 1920: 349–363.

[4] Head H, Holmes G. Studies in neurology. London: Frowde/Stodder and Houghton 1920

[5] Price D. Psychological mechanisms of pain and analgesia. Seattle: IASP Press 1999

[6] Melzack R, Wall P. The challenge of pain. London: Penguin 1996

[7] Melzack R. From the gate to the neuromatrix. Pain 1999; (Supplement 6):S121–S126

[8] Wall P. The gate control theory of pain mechanisms. A re-examination and re-statement. Brain 1978; 101:1–18

[9] Melzack R, Wall P. The challenge of pain. London: Penguin 1996

[10] Basbaum A, Dubner R, Fields H, McMahon S, Mendell L, Woolf C. A tribute to Patrick D. Wall. Pain 1999; (Supplement 6)

[11] Melzack R, Coderre T, Katz J, Vaccarino A. Central neuroplasticity and pathological pain. Annals of the New York Academy of Sciences 2001; 933:157–174

[12] Kandel E, Siegelbaum S. Synaptic integration. In: Kandel E, Schwartz J, Jessell T, eds. Principles of neural science. New York: McGraw-Hill 2000: 207–228

[13] Sims J. The mechanism of acupuncture analgesia: a review. Complement Ther Med 1997; (5):102–111

[14] Ready L, Edwards W. Management of acute pain: a practical guide. Seattle: IASP Publications 2001

[15] Pockett S. Spinal cord synaptic plasticity and chronic pain. Anesth Analg 1995; 80:173–179

[16] Doubell T, Mannion R, Woolf C. The dorsal horn: state-dependent sensory processing, plasticity and the generation of pain. In: Wall P, ed. Textbook of pain. Edinburgh: Churchill Livingstone 1999: 165–182

[17] Kandel E. Cellular mechanisms of learning and the biological basis of individuality. In: Kandel E, Schwartz J, Jessell T, eds. Principles of neural science. New York: McGraw-Hill, 2000: 1247–1279

[18] Moseley G. Evidence for a direct relationship between cognitive and physical change during an education intervention in people with chronic low back pain. European Journal of Pain 2004; 8:139–146

[19] Moseley G. Combined physiotherapy and education is efficacious for chronic low back pain. Australian Journal of Physiotherapy 2002; 48:297–302

[20] Woolf C. The dorsal horn: state-dependent sensory processing and the generation of pain. In: Wall P, ed. Textbook of pain. Edinburgh: Churchill Livingstone, 1994: 101–112

[21] Mannion R, Doubell T, Coggeshall R, Woolf C. Collateral sprouting of injured primary afferent A-fibres into the superficial dorsal horn of the adult rat spinal cord after topical capsaicin treatment to the sciatic nerve. J Neurosci 1996; 16:5189–5195

[22] Hansson P, Kinnman E. Unmasking mechanisms of peripheral neuropathic pain in a clinical perspective. Pain Rev 1996; 3:4272–4292

[23] Woolf C, Salter M. Neuronal plasticity: increasing the gain in pain. Science 2000; 288:1765–1768

[24] Korr I, ed. The neurobiologic mechanisms in manipulative therapy. New York: Plenum Press 1978

[25] Sarkar S, Aziz Q, Woolf C, Hobson A, Thompson D. Contribution of central sensitization to the development of non-cardiac chest pain. Lancet 2000; 356:1154–1159

[26] Coutinho S, Su X, Sengupta J, Gebhart G. Role of sensitized pelvic nerve afferents from the inflamed rat colon in the maintenance of visceral hyperalgesia. In: Sandkühler J, Bromm B, Gebhart G, eds. Nervous system plasticity and chronic pain. Amsterdam: Elsevier 2000: 375–387

[27] Arendt-Nielsen L, Laursen R, Drewes A. Referred pain as an indicator for neural plasticity. In: Sandkühler J, Bromm B, Gebhart G, eds. Nervous system plasticity and chronic pain. Amsterdam: Elsevier 2000: 344–356

[28] Cervero F, Laird J. Visceral pain. Lancet 1999; 353:2145–2148

[29] McMahon S. Are there fundamental differences in the peripheral mechanisms of visceral and somatic pain? Behav Brain Sci 1997; 20:381–391

[30] Ness T. Historical and clinical perspectives of visceral pain. In: Gebhart G, ed. Visceral pain. Seattle: IASP Press 1995: 3–24

[31] van Cranenburgh B. Pijn – vanuit een neurowetenschappelijk perspectief (Pain from a neuroscientific perspective). Maarssen: Elsevier Gezondheidszorg 2000

[32] Ness T, Gebhart G. Visceral pain: a review of experimental studies. Pain 1990; 41:167–234

[33] Laursen R, Graven-Nielsen T, Jensen T, Arendt-Nielsen L. The effect of compression and regional anaesthetic block on referred pain intensity in humans. Pain 1999; (80,1):2257–2263

[34] Sinclair D. Mechanisms of cutaneous sensation, 2nd edn. Oxford: Oxford University Press 1981

[35] Baldry P. Acupuncture, trigger points and musculoskeletal pain, 2nd edn. Edinburgh: Churchill Livingstone 1993

[36] Mann F. Reinventing acupuncture. A new concept of ancient medicine, 2nd edn. Oxford: Butterworth Heinemann 2000

[37] Mulligan B. Manual therapy – 'NAGS', 'SNAGS', 'PRPs' etc. Wellington: Plain View 1989

[38] Piët J, Sachs J, Sachs-Piët I. Bindweefselmassage, 4th edn. Lochem, De Tijdstroom, 1989

[39] Holey L. Connective tissue manipulation – Towards a scientific rationale. Physiotherapy 1995; 81:12

[40] Jänig W. Neurologische grondslagen. In: Piët J, Sachs J, Sachs-Piët I, eds. Bindweefselmassage. Lochem: De Tijdstroom, 1989: 22–61

[41] Bradnam L. Western acupuncture point selection: a scientific clinical reasoning model. Journal of the Acupuncture Association of Chartered Physiotherapists 2002; 21–29

[42] Moseley G. Unravelling the barriers to reconceptualisation of the problem in chronic pain: the actual and perceived ability of patients and health professionals to understand the neurophysiology. J Pain 2003; 7:4184–4189

[43] Barker R, Barasi S, Neal M. Neuroscience at a glance. Oxford: Blackwell Science, 2000

[44] Kandel E. Nerve cells and behaviour. In: Kandel E, Schwartz J, Jessell T, eds. Principles of neural science. New York: McGraw-Hill, 2000: 19–35

[45] Alberts B, Johnson A, Lewis J, Raff M, Roberts K, Walter P. Molecular biology of the cell, 4th edn, New York: Garland Science 2002

[46] Travell J, Rinzler S. The myofascial genesis of pain. Trigger areas in myofascial structures can maintain pain indefinitely. Postgraduate Medicine 1952; 11:425–434

[47] Ferner H, Staubesand J. Sobotta atlas of human anatomy, 10th edn. München: Urban and Schwartzenberg 1982

[48] van Cranenburgh B. Neurowetenschappen – een overzicht. Maarssen: Elsevier/De Tijdstroom 1999

[49] Cheng X. Chinese acupuncture and moxibustion. Beijing: Foreign Languages Press 1990

[50] Gardner E, Martin J, Jessell T. The bodily senses. In: Kandel E, Schwartz J, Jessell T, eds. Principles of neural science. New York: McGraw-Hill 2000: 430–450

[51] de Morree J. Dynamiek van het menselijk bindweefsel. Functie, beschadiging en herstel. Utrecht: Bohn, Scheltema and Holkema 1989

The not-so-sympathetic nervous system

A sunset will be created for you. I shall insist on it. However, in my wisdom I shall wait until the circumstances are favourable.

ANTOINE DE SAINT-EXUPÉRY, THE LITTLE PRINCE

INTRODUCTION

Pain may be an indication that something is wrong with the body. However, it has become clear in the previous chapters how sometimes the nervous system rather than the tissues is responsible for generating pain. An interesting feature of peripheral and central neurogenic pains is that the brain persists in interpreting them as arising from the tissues (Fig. 3.1). As a result the response of the nervous system to ongoing pain is the same, regardless of its origin.

Injury and pain may trigger what is often referred to as the *stress response*, or the *fight or flight response*, a way of preparing the body to deal with an immediate threat.[1] Multiple body systems are prepared to either get out of the unpleasant or dangerous situation, or to face the music and fight. This response is mediated by the autonomic nervous system and the hormonal system. In patients, it may manifest as agitation and the emotional and physical drive to find a cure.

While the body's potential for action is maximized by the fight or flight response, its restorative processes are slowed down or halted. Nutrition, rest and recovery are not a priority in a threatening situation, so they are put on hold until it is safe to drop one's guard. In the case of animals, this is a state that does not persist for very long. When an animal needs to get out of a sticky situation, the outcome is usually straightforward: either the animal escapes or it is killed. The fight or flight response facilitates the burst of energy and activity required to deal with the acute situation. However, for human beings a threatening situation may persist over a long period. After a while, the stress response becomes maladaptive, because it wears out the body's resources. The body pays the price for the persistent lack of restoration; the mind for not settling down.

One of the reasons that stress can become a more persistent problem for humans is the fact that the stress response does not differentiate between physical and psychological threats. For example, the prospect of job redundancy prepares a person's body for action, even though no physical threat is present. Similarly, patients with persistent pain may be under no physical threat whatsoever, but still show a marked autonomic response.

The importance of the stress response for therapists dealing with persistent pain is twofold. First, persistent pain is often perceived by the patient as an ongoing threat and may be associated with increased vigilance, psychological and muscular tension and exhaustion as a result. Second, the tissues may not be able to respond to manual therapy if the patient's autonomic and hormonal status does not allow it. For example, if the *catecholamines* adrenaline and noradrenaline prevent peripheral blood vessels from responding to treatments designed to improve circulation, the intended facilitation of the healing process may not take place (Fig. 2.7). In addition, cortisol reduces the availability of amino acids that are needed for tissue healing.

The poor capillary response combined with the impaired potential for tissue repair in patients with stress can undermine musculoskeletal treatments. Tissue effects such as improved circulation, formation of functional collagen and changes in the number of contractile elements in a muscle all rely on the cooperation of the autonomic and endocrine systems. Treatment may therefore have to be a two-staged approach, in which the body is enabled to allow healing of its tissues before the tissue problems themselves are addressed. Physical therapists often address these issues implicitly by using explanation, reassurance and relaxation, but these approaches are not always incorporated in the clinical reasoning process.

This chapter discusses various physiological components of the stress response and circumstances that may act as triggers. Signs and symptoms suggestive of maladaptive autonomic and endocrine involvement are listed and followed by recommended therapeutic strategies. The psychological elements of these strategies are mentioned, but they are dealt with in detail in Chapter 6.

Finally, Complex Regional Pain Syndrome, Type 1 is described. This is one of the few disorders encountered in musculoskeletal practice with signs of malfunction of the sympathetic nervous system. However, the mechanisms that generate symptoms are far from clear[2] and the involvement of the sympathetic nervous system is the subject of ongoing scientific dispute.[3] The available knowledge is reviewed, together with diagnostic criteria and recommendations for treatment.

THE HYPOTHALAMIC–PITUITARY–ADRENAL (HPA) AXIS

Situations and events that are perceived as threatening trigger the arousal associated with the so-called stress response, which is mediated by the processes represented in Figure 5.1.[1] The hypothalamus activates the sympathetic nerves, which release *noradrenaline* (also known as *norepinephrine*) from their terminals, thereby affecting the viscera and somatic tissues. The sympathetic fibres that terminate in the adrenal medulla stimulate the release of *adrenaline* (also called *epinephrine*) and noradrenaline into the circulation, leading to wide-

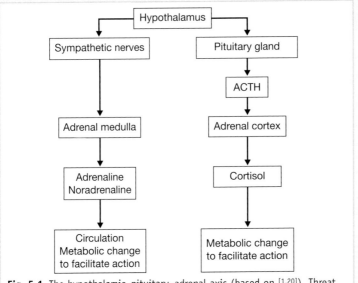

Fig. 5.1 The hypothalamic–pituitary–adrenal axis (based on [1,20]). Threat activates the hypothalamus, which in turn stimulates the sympathetic nervous system and the pituitary gland. This either directly or indirectly leads to the release of adrenaline, noradrenaline and cortisol and affects circulation and metabolism.

spread sympathetic effects. The sympathetic response therefore has a neural as well as a *humoral* or *endocrine* element.

The exact effects of noradrenaline and adrenaline depend on the distribution of different adrenal receptors in the tissues (Fig. 5.2). In the author's experience, many musculoskeletal therapists are aware of the visceral, but not the musculoskeletal effects of sympathetic activity, because this is the emphasis reinforced by physiology texts. This is unfortunate, because the effects on the somatic tissues are of greater

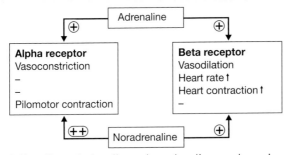

Fig. 5.2 The effects of adrenaline and noradrenaline on adrenergic receptors most relevant for the musculoskeletal system.[1] Noradrenaline has a stronger effect on alpha receptors than on beta receptors, while adrenaline's action is equal for both. The exact effect depends on the distribution of these receptors.

Table 5.1 Effects of sympathetic stimulation on somatic tissues and circulation (after [1])

Blood pressure	Acute increase due to increased heart effort and vascular resistance
Arterioles of skin, muscle	Constriction by alpha receptors Dilation by beta 2 and cholinergic receptors
Composition of blood	Increased glucose and lipids
Basal metabolism	Increased
Pilo-erector muscles	Contraction
Skeletal muscle	Increased breakdown of glycogen to form glucose
Fat cells	Breakdown of fats into fatty acids

importance in clinical practice. The effects most relevant for somatic effects are summarized in Table 5.1. The parasympathetic nervous system *does not affect any of the tissues treated by musculoskeletal clinicians*. It is therefore not relevant for the current discussion.

In addition to activating the sympathetic nerves, the hypothalamus stimulates the pituitary gland to release *adrenocorticotropic hormone (ACTH)*, which regulates another part of the adrenal gland, the *adrenal medulla*. The most important hormone released by the adrenal medulla is cortisol, which has a wide range of effects on energy release and inflammation.

The body's most effective way of releasing the energy required for the fight-or-flight response is the breakdown of glucose. Cortisol increases the blood glucose levels by stimulating its production from amino acids and fat, while simultaneously reducing its use by most cells. It also reduces the storage of proteins in the cells and facilitates the release of their constituent amino acids into the circulation, thereby increasing the potential for producing glucose. The use of amino acids for the formation of collagen fibres is reduced. Finally, it mobilizes fatty acids that can be used for energy release if glucose cannot be used.

Apart from the effects that cortisol has on metabolic processes, there are effects on inflammation. Immediately after tissue damage, cortisol can block progression to the inflammatory stage (see Ch. 2). If the inflammatory process has already started, cortisol speeds up its resolution.[1] One could say that the release of cortisol in an emergency enables the body to either put inflammation and repair on hold, or to get over them as soon as possible. These processes are not a priority for fight or flight.

The most primitive nervous system has a string of nociceptive inputs and motor outputs, linked by a reflex arc (Fig. 5.3). The organism could be a worm, capable of withdrawing from potentially damaging stimuli. An element of sophistication is introduced by the addition of a central regulating centre or brain and a sensory system for non-noxious stimuli (see also Ch.2, p. 17).

The chance of survival is increased by the organism's ability to rally all its resources quickly, in order to either fight or escape. Sympathetic nerves form at a segmental level, going out with the motor neurones. Their activity is influenced by the input from segmental afferents and controls circulation and metabolism, so that energy can be made available and utilized quickly and effectively. In addition, the hypothalamus forms a central regulation centre for sympathetic activity. It also stimulates the release of adrenaline by the adrenal glands, which further facilitates a general response.

With a sophisticated sensory and motor system in place and the ability to maximize the ability to respond, evolution can begin to concentrate on maximizing the organism's potential to recover, replenish and repair. The brain stem extends the vagal nerve directly to the internal organs of chest and abdomen, and forms a sacral regulating centre for pelvic organs. This so-called *parasympathetic* system (literally 'alongside the sympathetic') facilitates metabolic function and in some cases counteracts sympathetic action. This enables the organism to invoke restorative processes quickly and maximize them, rather than having to wait for the adrenal and sympathetic effects to die away and allow recovery to happen by default.

Not directly related to the development of different types of nervous system, is the development of limbs. The type of spinal cord described above, has an equal number of neurones arising from each segment. However, as the limbs developed more space was required for their sensory and motor neurones. Because the spine did not allow much spinal cord expansion, the cell bodies of sympathetic nerves were forced to migrate to areas where only relatively small dorsal and ventral horn were needed.[1] In human beings, sympathetic control for the arms stems from the mid- to upper thoracic segments, while the legs are controlled from the lower thoracic and upper lumbar segments. Sensory and motor neurones are located in the lower cervical and lumbosacral regions.

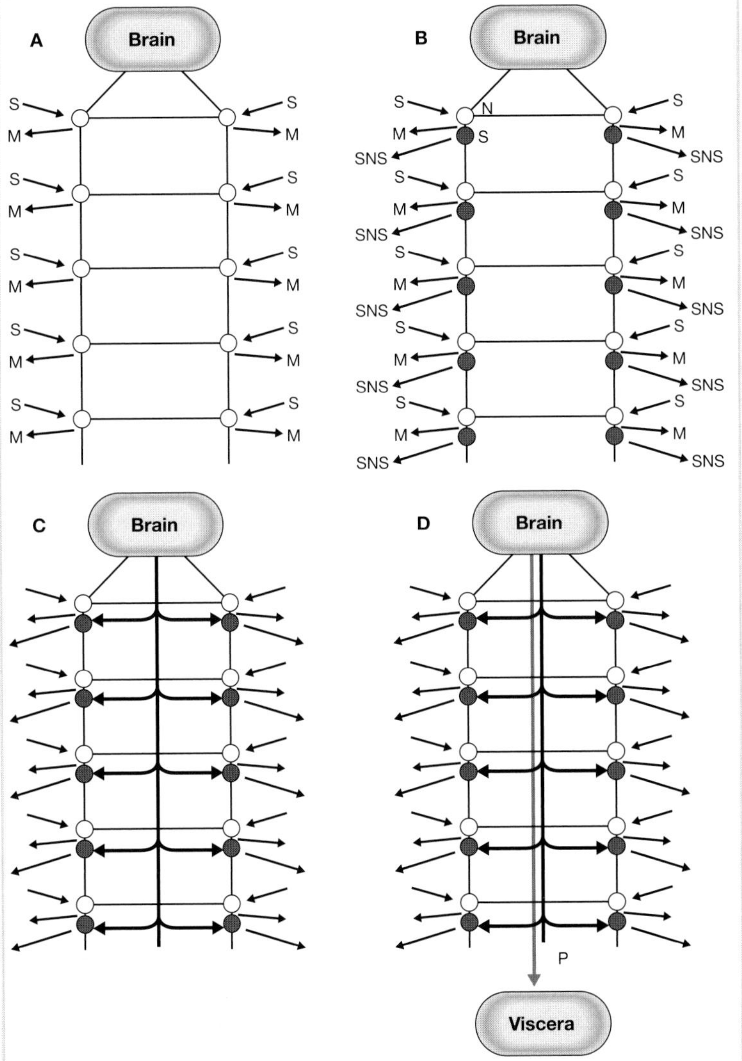

Fig. 5.3 Development of the nervous system in evolution. **A.** The primitive nervous system of a worm consists of interconnected nodes N, which receive sensory input S and react to noxious stimuli with a motor response M. **B.** Each segment develops a sympathetic centre S that enables a more effective reaction to threatening stimuli via regulation of circulation and glucose production. **C.** The sympathetic centres are regulated centrally by the brain. **D.** Optimal regulation of restorative processes is achieved by a direct link from the brain to the internal organs. This is the parasympathetic nervous system P.

Box 5.2 Selye's General Adaptation Syndrome[1,4–6]

In the first half of the 20th century, the medical student Hans Selye noticed characteristics that unified many patients regardless of their exact medical problem: they looked and felt ill. Rather than focusing on a particular branch of medicine, he became interested in the signs and symptoms underlying illness. Several years later, he was conducting research on rats that were subjected to various trying circumstances such as cold, injections or hard exercise. He noticed that these rats produced stomach ulcers and developed enlarged adrenal glands.

Selye went on to develop his ideas into the General Adaptation Syndrome. This is divided into three stages:

- Physical or psychological trauma triggers the alarm reaction briefly discussed in the introduction to this chapter.
- If the stressful circumstance persists, the organism may get used to it. It adapts by making its immune system work harder than usual and suppressing the effects of stress.
- Eventually, the body reaches the limits of its capacity to resist stress, possibly because another stressing event occurs. Organ systems are no longer able to cope and the immune system is depleted.

Selye decided that high blood pressure, gastric ulcers and other conditions were diseases of adaptation. His ideas became very popular with the public, who recognized his model of stress in their own lives. However, the scientific and medical community was more resistant and had reason to be so. Selye had published his views before they were peer reviewed. This scuppered the chance of research on unbiased subjects. Selye had also created a trend of describing stress as if it were a well-defined entity, like a virus or a chemical, whereas in reality it could be more accurately described as an interaction between a person and his environment. This led to the formulation of stress tables, which gave a rating to each type of life event such as moving house, death of a relative or getting married. It is clear that the response to each of these events is determined by the circumstances, the culture and the individual; moving is unlikely to upset a nomadic tribesman.

Despite these and other shortcomings, Selye's work made some important contributions to science.[7] It made the relevance of the pituitary–adrenal system clear and introduced the idea that adaptation could be a cause of disease. It also provided an explanation for non-specific diseases that were previously considered idiopathic.

THE LONG-TERM EFFECTS OF AROUSAL

As outlined above, in the face of a threat it is advantageous to mobilize all one's energy resources and prepare all defence systems for immediate and vigorous action. Because the resources are finite, this necessitates putting processes with less urgency on hold. While this can be a successful way of dealing with a temporary situation, prolonged activation of the HPA axis has effects that are detrimental to the person. Hans Selye pioneered activation of this system as a cause of disease (Box 5.2).

Cortisol reduces the availability of amino acids for the repair of the soft tissues. The half-life of collagen is about 350–500 days, so in 18 months or less half of the body's collagen is replaced.[8] If the amino acids needed for this regenerative process are not available, the quality of muscles, ligaments and tendons reduces over time. Therapies aimed at stimulating soft tissue repair are likely to be less effective in this situation. Through high levels of cortisol, pain-induced stress can therefore reduce the body's capacity to respond to treatment and make it more prone to further injury. This may make fear of (re-) injury a self-fulfilling prophecy (Fig. 5.4 and see also Ch. 6). Ronald Melzack points out that some forms of chronic pain may occur as a result of cumulative destructive effect of cortisol on muscle, bone and neural tissue.[9]

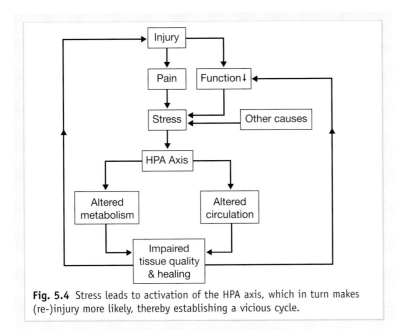

Fig. 5.4 Stress leads to activation of the HPA axis, which in turn makes (re-)injury more likely, thereby establishing a vicious cycle.

Persistently high activity levels of the sympathetic nervous system, also called the *sympathetic tone*, prevent the circulation from returning to a state that allows tissue repair. Not only does cortisol reduce the availability of materials, a circulatory response inhibited by the superimposition of sympathetic activity means that these meagre supplies don't reach the tissues that need them.

The therapist who finds several indications that a patient's body may be demonstrating the consequences of long-term stress is justified in addressing the HPA axis before turning to the treatment of specific tissues. After all, this system can override or interfere with the capacity of any tissue to respond to musculoskeletal treatment. Without its cooperation, treatment aimed at promoting healing and repair is likely to fail (Fig. 5.4).

FUNCTIONAL ANATOMY OF THE SYMPATHETIC NERVOUS SYSTEM

The following section is based on references [1,10,11].

Many texts dealing with the physiology of the sympathetic nervous system present the reader with a diagram of the spinal cord, paravertebral ganglia and viscera (Fig. 5.5). Lines indicating nerves run from the thoracic region of the spinal cord to the *paravertebral ganglia*. Other nerves link the paravertebral ganglia with the viscera and eyes. The musculoskeletal therapist looking at this picture could be forgiven for wondering what its relevance is to manual therapy, because no somatic target is present. Usually a lengthy table, cataloguing an impressive list of sympathetic effects on each target organ, follows the diagram. Only a tiny, frequently overlooked section men-

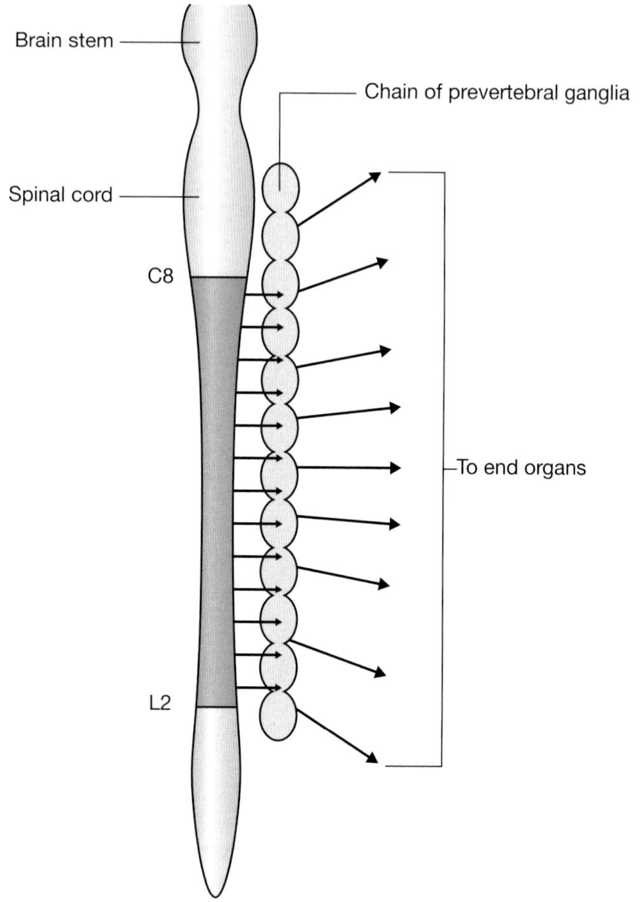

Fig. 5.5 Simplified diagram of the sympathetic nervous system (based on [1,47]).Pre-ganglionic nerves (short arrows) go from the spinal cord to the paravertebral ganglia, where they link with post-ganglionic nerves (long arrows). These nerves go to end organs in viscera, sense organs and somatic structures.

Brain stem

Chain of prevertebral ganglia

Spinal cord

C8

To end organs

L2

tions the musculoskeletal system and skin. This discrepancy belies the fact that sympathetic nerves influence every musculoskeletal tissue in the body.

This section describes the parts of the autonomic nervous system most relevant for physical therapists. The parasympathetic nervous system is not discussed, because it does not affect any musculoskeletal structures. Readers interested in parasympathetic function or sympathetic effects on viscera and cranium are advised to turn to standard texts, some of which are listed in the reference list at the end of this chapter.[1,10,11]

Sympathetic outflow to musculoskeletal structures consists of *preganglionic* and *postganglionic nerves* (Fig. 5.6). The cell bodies of the sympathetic preganglionic fibres are situated in the lateral intermediate horn of the spinal cord, similar to the cell bodies of motor neurones in the ventral horn. Preganglionic nerves are short, because they only go from the spinal cord to a ganglion to the side of the spine. All levels of the spine including cervical and lumbosacral have

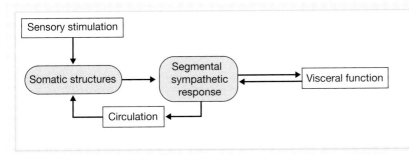

Fig. 5.6 Somatosympathetic reflex (after [48]). Stimulation of somatic sensory nerves terminating in the dorsal horn influences the sympathetic nerves originating from the same spinal level. This in turn has an effect on the viscera. The opposite effect i.e. visceral stimulation that influences somatic structures, can also take place.

ganglia, forming a long string either side of the vertebral bodies called the sympathetic chain.

There is considerable divergence in sympathetic outflow, because preganglionic nerves may go to several ganglia. Sympathetic neurones supplying the cervical and lumbosacral spinal nerves do so by synapsing at the relevant levels. Preganglionic nerves may synapse with more than one postganglionic neurone, which can outnumber them by a ratio of 200:1 in some cases.[10] It is therefore unrealistic to expect a very specific segmental effect from for example the manipulation of a vertebra or the release of a paravertebral muscle.

Postganglionic nerves carry action potentials from the sympathetic ganglia to the target tissues. They end in a great number of varicosities containing vesicles with transmitter chemicals. Most sympathetic vesicles contain noradrenaline, although those innervating the sweat glands, piloerector muscles and some blood vessels contain acetylcholine. Transmitter is released when depolarization opens calcium channels, creating a calcium flow into the nerve. This process is similar to the release of neurotransmitter in the synapse, as described in the previous chapter. An overview of the effects is given in Table 5.1.

Output of sympathetic neurones in the lateral intermediate horn is regulated in two ways. Central regulation is performed by the hypothalamus, which forms a regulatory centre that receives sensory information from almost the entire body, including chemoreceptors. It controls several homeostatic processes by changing the activity of the autonomic nervous system and the endocrine system if the incoming information does not match the internal standards. In addition, it motivates behavioural changes to facilitate the adaptation. For instance, if a change in body temperature is needed, endocrine and autonomic function can be changed to alter metabolism, circulation and sweat production. At the same time, the person will get the urge to seek a more moderate environment.

Hypothalamic regulation is usually described as adaptation of the internal environment of the body in response to a changing external world. This is suggestive of a passive process, independent of the mind. A different interpretation is that the hypothalamus tunes the body to facilitate whatever the person's intentions and emotions demand. Activities (including rest!) are instigated by the mental and emotional mind, and homeostatic processes maximize the body's potential to do what the mind dictates. This adaptation makes the body like a car engine, which can be changed from an efficient city model to a racing engine or an agricultural workhorse at the flick of a switch.

The second regulatory process is of a segmental nature. Sensory neurones from the tissues form synaptic links with the sympathetic nerves in the lateral intermediate horn. This explains the appearance of cutaneous zones because of noxious sensory input from a visceral structure as described by Head (see Treatment approaches in Ch. 4, p. 75). It may also explain how specific treatments of those zones provide sensory input which alters sympathetic regulation of the affected organ (Fig. 5.6).[12] The effect of cutaneous stimulation of either the sacral or thoracolumbar segments on micturition can easily be verified by the reader.

Sato and Schmidt described how brief stimulation of myelinated afferents type II and III could evoke a temporary increase in segmental sympathetic activity, followed by a reduction.[13] However, a later review by the same authors suggests that most of the sympathetic response is excitatory, especially when the stimulation is of a noxious nature.[14] Interestingly, the sensation created during treatment for visceral pathology with acupuncture or CTM is often suggestive of A delta stimulation and is usually followed by a reduction in signs and symptoms associated with sympathetic activity. Although this may hint at a segmental response, the fact that these treatments are often followed by drowsiness, lack of concentration and occasional *vaso-vagal reaction* (fainting as a result of vasodilation, sometimes seen in emotional reactions)[15,16] suggests significant effects on the brain. Evidence of well-defined segmental sympathetic reflexes that enable the clinician to predict the response to a given stimulus is as yet unavailable.

SUBJECTIVE EXAMINATION OF THE HPA AXIS

The aim of this element of the examination is to find signs that are suggestive of ongoing activation of the HPA system, or in other words signs of adrenergic and adrenocortical effects. Every attempt must be made to verify subjective signs in the objective examination.

General symptoms

Because the effects of the HPA system are widespread and non-specific, a single finding can never be significant on its own. Rather, the clinician has to find whether a collection of symptoms forms a pattern (see Box 5.3 for an overview). For example, frequent gastric upsets can have a multitude of causes. However, if the patient also complains of sleeplessness, lack of concentration and nervousness, the gastric symptoms become part of a pattern that may well be related to stress.

Box 5.3 General symptoms of HPA overactivity[49]

- Palpitations
- Hyperventilation can manifest in a variety of ways, many of which are not obviously of a respiratory nature. The Nijmegen questionnaire can help to objectify the clinician's impression[50]
- Nausea
- Light headedness
- Lack of concentration
- Lack of libido
- Lack of appetite
- Variations in blood pressure
- Hyperhidrosis
- Disorganized behaviour

A word of caution concerns the label of stress. A wide range of factors influences the hypothalamus, pituitary and adrenal glands. They have a range of effects, which in turn have feedback systems to the HPA. It is important that the clinician tries to find which elements have led to the current symptomatology and which are involved in maintaining it. Identification of these elements enables the clinician to formulate a therapeutic strategy, whereas the use of the blanket term stress is more likely to get the patient unjustifiably written off as 'not for manual therapy'.

Segmentally related symptoms

The overview of segmental relationships between visceral and somatic structures can help to decide whether the sympathetic nervous system is likely to be an important factor. It must be remembered that the sympathetic nervous system is rather diffuse. It is therefore possible to decide on a spinal region of importance, not on a single segment.

The clinician is advised to ask the patient whether any visceral symptoms have been present. If symptoms of a particular organ system are expected, the patient may need to be pressed. For example, he may have adapted to a mild stomach dysfunction several years before by avoiding certain foods. This dietary change has now become routine and is no longer thought of, and neither is the stomach problem. The patient may only remember it when asked whether he eats everything, or whether certain foods cause a reaction.

The following symptom complexes are suggestive of segmental mediation:

1. Lumbosacral region
   a. Circulatory problems of the lower limbs
   b. Poor healing of the lower limbs
   c. Lumbosacral and sacroiliac pain and stiffness
   d. Bladder symptoms: cystitis, frequency, incontinence
   e. Symptoms of the reproductive system: period problems, pain, impotence
   f. Bowel symptoms: constipation; diarrhoea; Irritable Bowel Syndrome (IBS). (Note: IBS is considered to be a functional bowel disorder, not associated with any visceral pathology but mediated by neural mechanisms.[17,18] Therefore, the diagnosis of IBS can only be made by exclusion, i.e after a negative full examination by a gastroenterologist.)
2. Thoracolumbar region
   a. Pain and stiffness of the upper lumbar and mid to lower thoracic region, lower ribs and hypochondriac region
   b. Gastric symptoms: loss of appetite, avoidance of certain foods, ulceration, acidity, indigestion
   c. Symptoms of liver and gallbladder: intolerance of fatty foods and alcohol

d. Irritation of the diaphragm and peritoneum can stimulate the phrenic nerve (C2–4) and create neck and shoulder symptoms

e. Kidney-related symptoms: kidney stones, loin pain, bladder symptoms.

3. Thoracic region

a. Chest symptoms: tightness, pain, movement restriction

b. Shoulder symptoms: pain and stiffness of scapulae and shoulder joints

c. Cardiac symptoms: palpitations, fast fatigue on exertion, oedema of feet and ankles

d. Respiratory symptoms: shortness of breath, frequent coughing, phlegm, bronchitis, asthma.

4. Cervicothoracic region

a. Cervical symptoms: pain, movement restriction

b. Cranial symptoms: headaches, blurred vision, sinusitis, dizziness

c. Shoulder symptoms: pain, stiffness.

Sometimes a patient describes an empirical link between symptoms, for example a recurring cystitis that is always associated with a particular type of headache. This is suggestive of the presence of a central influence. Patients can be asked whether they have observed a similarity in timing or trigger of seemingly disparate symptoms, to form an impression of the most likely therapeutic target. The more widespread and interactive the symptoms are, the more likely it is that a more general or central approach needs to precede localized treatment.

A word of warning concerns the interpretation of a complex of symptoms. The symptoms created by any pathology can both interact with pre-existing symptoms and affect the HPA system. Treatment of symptoms without addressing their cause can be dangerous. If there is any doubt about underlying pathology, the patient must be referred to either their General Practitioner or an appropriate specialist.

OBJECTIVE EXAMINATION OF HPA FUNCTION

The signs in Box 5.4 are suggestive of persistently high levels of adrenal and sympathetic activity and are adapted from Bernards.[19]

TREATMENT OF HPA OVERACTIVITY

The preceding three chapters have dealt with pain problems related to influences, from local through regional to central. The signs and symptoms that are the subject of this chapter relate to body regions, groups of segments and systems affecting the whole body. Many patients with persistent pain have signs and symptoms that do not relate to a single nerve or tissue, often to the frustration of both therapist and patient. These patients present with pains and trophic changes in several segmentally related structures or even the whole body. When this is the case, the central influence is likely to need treatment before the more local issues are addressed (Fig. 5.7 and Box 5.5).

Box 5.4 Signs of persistently high levels of adrenal and sympathetic activity

Skin
- Discoloration: pale, blue, grey
- Reduction in temperature
- Reduction in capillary refill
- Increased sweat production
- Pilo-erection
- Reduction in pliability
- Increased adherence to the fascia
- 'Thicker' consistency
- Increased resistance to stretch
- Sensory changes: hyperaesthesia, hyperalgesia, allodynia

Muscle
- Increased resistance to stretch
- Reduction in length
- Increased muscle tone
- Increased fatiguability
- Frequent cramps
- Discomfort or pain on stretch and/or contraction

Joint
- Stiff end feel
- Reduction of range of movement in a capsular pattern
- Discomfort or pain at end of range

Nerve
- Increased resistance to neural tension tests
- Discomfort or pain when stretched

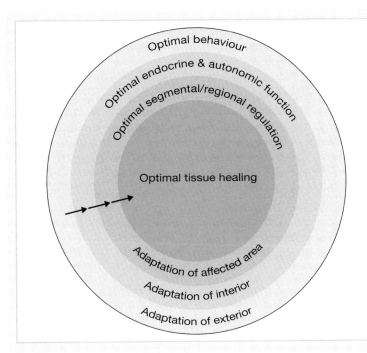

Fig. 5.7 Order of importance in treating persistent musculoskeletal signs and symptoms, in the presence of segmental, regional or general trophic changes. If general issues of behaviour and internal regulation are not sub-optimal, the healing response may be impaired.

Box 5.5 A patient with poor tissue healing

A patient presents with an old inversion injury of the right ankle. The injury was incurred 3 months ago but refuses to improve. The patient is extremely worried that a fracture may have been missed when he presented at casualty immediately after the injury. He is also concerned that he may lose his job.

Examination of the ankle confirms a sprain of the anterior talofibular ligament. Both feet are cold to the touch, suggesting less than optimal regulation of the circulation by the sympathetic and/or adrenal system. It is already clear to the therapist that the patient's overall HPA activity is raised by stress regarding the injury and its consequences. He also establishes that there may be a segmental pattern, because the patient has a history of recurrent low backache and has experienced an increased frequency of micturition in the last 6 weeks.

The therapist addresses stress and the HPA axis by giving a detailed explanation of the diagnosis and its consequences. He acquires the X-rays and shows the patient that no fracture is present. He also gives detailed advice regarding the regular use of ice and exercise. This does not only have a physical effect, but also focuses the patient's mind on adaptive behaviour instead of flitting from one potential worry to another. The therapist explores the nature of the patient's work. Together with the patient, he devises strategies that put the patient in control and reduce the concerns about job loss.

Following principle of overflow, which suggests that contralateral limbs affect each other, the patient is taught an aerobic exercise regime for the unaffected leg. Later, stretching exercises for the lumbosacral region and the gluteal and thigh muscles of the affected leg are included. These exercises provide normal and normalizing input into the affected segments in order to affect sympathetic activity, without aggravating the ankle or worrying the patient. These exercises are complemented by manual techniques designed to provide further sensory input into the affected segment.

As a result of the therapeutic approach that targets the interlinked elements of stress, perceived control, central and segmental regulation of sympathetic activity, the patient's function improves. Bladder function and circulation in the feet normalize. It is now that the therapist deems the time right to start local treatment for the ankle. Previously, pain caused by the treatment would have alarmed the patient even more. Poor circulation caused by sympathetic overactivity would have made it difficult for the tissues to respond to therapy. Physiotherapy intervention can be effective, but the circumstances have to be right.

This approach works from general to specific, from central to peripheral. The reason is that the influence of the HPA axis affects the ability of the person to respond to therapy, from both a psychological and a physical perspective.

An (over) activated HPA system brings the person into a state of non-specific arousal. Body and mind are ready for action, whatever that action will turn out to be. Either this arousal will settle when the threat is removed, or it will be used to deal with the threat. If nothing is resolved, the body's capacity to relax, replenish and heal is likely to reduce. One of the first things a therapist should therefore do is to assess the patient and explain exactly what the findings mean. This is an essential ingredient of an approach that aims to reduce non-specific arousal. Involving the patient and giving specific exercises and tasks aid this further. By doing this, the therapist enables the patient to focus their arousal on specific targets. This can help to reduce anxiety and overall HPA activity.

- Some patients are helped enormously by relaxation exercises. Some therapists may wish to prescribe a specific regime. Bookshops and shops focused on spiritual and mental wellbeing usually sell tapes and CDs with guided relaxation exercises. Some of the contacts at the back of this book send these by mail order. Neil Berry's CD (see Appendix 7) contains a relaxation section, but talks the patient through principles of pain management as well.
- Although relaxation can be beneficial, it has to be introduced when the patient is ready for it. For example, it makes no sense to try to calm the patient prior to reassurance regarding the diagnosis. If the patient has genuine concerns, relaxation can be misplaced.
- Relaxation exercises are not the most natural way to relax for some people. For some, the distraction offered by vigorous exercise and the relaxation that naturally follows exertion may be more beneficial than lying still on a mat. It is up to the therapist to discover what method suits the patient best.
- If a part of the body cannot be exercised because of pain or limitation, the effects of the non-specific arousal can be used to exercise every other body part. Autonomic activity naturally goes down after physical exertion, so exercise may reduce the impact of stress on the body. It also helps to maintain overall fitness and resilience.
- If patients have little or no experience with exercise, they may need help in discovering what form of exercise suits them. It may be possible to establish a network of local exercise teachers, swimming instructors and meditation facilitators who allow patients to have a trial session.
- It may be necessary to explore specific stressors for the person, which may not stem from their symptoms. However, they are likely to maintain present pathology via the activation of the HPA system. Some therapists may be reluctant to explore this route, because they don't feel qualified to deal with mental and emotional trauma. Referral to a suitable professional is part of the next chapter, but is also discussed in some texts of interest for physical therapists.[20,21]

- The advice regarding exercise and treatment of structures related segmentally to the affected region applies here as well.

Some therapists claim that it is possible to affect the function of the nerves in the paravertebral ganglia by mobilizing the ribs. This makes little neural sense, because these ganglia move all the time with respiration and movement. Manual treatment of the thoracic region may well have sympathetic effects, but this is more likely to be due to stimulation of afferents and supraspinal responses. To draw an analogy, a computer mouse does not have any effect when its wire is mobilized, but only when its input device is manipulated.

CONTRIBUTION OF THE SYMPATHETIC NERVOUS SYSTEM TO PAIN

The notion of pain created by activity of the sympathetic nervous system is not without conceptual difficulties. Sympathetic nerves are *purely efferent* and in themselves are *not capable of generating pain*. The fact that they may share pathways with sensory nerves has led some to believe that sympathetic sensory nerves exist, but in reality there are no afferents dedicated to sympathetic function.[19] Noradrenaline and adrenaline are in themselves not algogenic. These catecholamines influence circulation, sweat production and a number of metabolic functions, none of which are normally associated with pain. The question is therefore whether this efferent system can generate pain, which is after all a sensory phenomenon.

Despite the absence of easily identifiable mechanisms explaining how the sympathetic nervous system can be involved in the generation of pain, there seems to be an empirical link in some patients.[22] In these patients, the painful region may show signs that are usually associated with sympathetic activity, such as changes in sweating and circulation, or the trophic state of the tissues. Few research trials supporting the idea of sympathetic involvement in the generation of pain exist, most of them uncontrolled.[22] However, some studies have demonstrated that patients may benefit from a sympathetic block, while noradrenaline is capable of stirring up the pain.[23] Despite this limited evidence, it is not clear what the underlying mechanisms are. Some historical models are discussed in Box 5.7.

The variety in manifestations of CRPS and the lack of agreement regarding its underlying mechanism is reflected in the number of names the condition has received over the years (Box 5.6). Current evidence is far from conclusive and a wide variety of causative mechanisms have been described (Table 5.2), suggesting that there may in fact be more than one mechanism underlying the manifestations of this syndrome. In addition to specific injuries and pathologies, there is evidence that immobilization alone can produce some of the characteristics associated with CRPS.[27] Animal studies have generated hypotheses regarding the influence of sympathetic activity on peripheral sensory nerves, but their applicability in humans is not always clear (Box 5.8).

Box 5.6 Some terms used for sympathetic pain syndromes (after [24,51]). This list is long but not exhaustive!

- Algo(neuro)dystrophy
- Causalgia
- Chronic traumatic oedema
- Complex regional pain disorder
- Neurodystrophy
- Pain-dysfunction syndrome
- Post-traumatic oedema
- Post-traumatic osteoporosis
- Post-traumatic pain syndrome
- Post-traumatic spreading neuralgia
- Reflex (sympathetic) dystrophy
- Shoulder–hand syndrome
- Südeck's atrophy
- Sympathalgia
- Sympathetic overdrive syndrome
- Traumatic arthritis

TABLE 5.2 Initiating events of CRPS The results of four studies have been pooled for a total of 778 patients.[24]

Trauma	
Blunt	32
Laceration	11
Fracture	21
Sprain	2
Nerve injury	1
Total trauma	67 %
Postoperative	
Carpal tunnel	6
Dupuytren's	4
Ganglion cyst	2
Other	2
Unspecified	5
Total post-op.	21 %
Burns	
Thermal	1
Electrical	1
Total burns	2 %
MI	2 %
Cerebral disease	1 %
Spinal cord injury	<1%
Other/unknown	5 %

Over the years, several theories have been proposed in an attempt to explain coupling between sympathetic and nociceptive activity.[24] The theory put forward by Lewis in the 1930s was based on the so-called axon reflex, the release of neuropeptides when C fibres are stimulated. These chemicals in turn have algogenic and vasodilatory effects (see Ch. 2, p. 23), which may explain the swelling, discoloration and local tenderness associated with some forms of CRPS. Although there is evidence that this peripheral mechanism plays a role,[25] it does not explain why sympathectomy can relieve pain.

Other theories involve the development of reflex loops. An example is the model put forward by Roberts (Fig. 5.8), based on evidence that sympathetic activity could affect the function of mechanoreceptors.[26] Mechanoreceptors can create pain when the WDR cells in the dorsal horn become sensitized by ongoing nociceptive activity (see Ch.4, p. 64). Roberts suggested that sympathetic activity could cause pain via mechanoreceptor stimulation, once central sensitization had developed. This mechanism can become self-perpetuating, because the sympathetic cells in the lateral intermediate horn are stimulated by nociceptive input. However, the fact that in many patients with the clinical manifestations of CRPS there is no evidence of sympathetic dysfunction, suggests that Roberts' model is incomplete.[22]

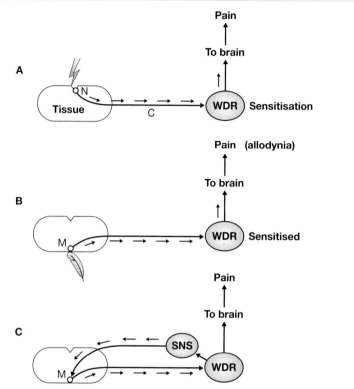

Fig. 5.8 A model of CRPS proposed by Roberts.[26] **A.** Ongoing stimulation of nociceptor N, for instance by tissue damage, leads to sensitization of a WDR cell. **B.** The sensitized WDR cell makes non-noxious stimulation of mechanoreceptors M painful (allodynia). **C.** Sympathetic (SNS) activation continues to activate mechanoreceptors in absence of peripheral stimulation. The resulting nociceptive activity maintains sympathetic tone in a vicious cycle.

Patients with CRPS may have generalized changes in sensory and motor function not explained by the peripheral innervation.[28] This suggests that the condition has a central component, a finding supported by a study that showed altered brain responses in CRPS patients.[29] Recently, exciting new evidence has been added to this hypothesis by demonstrating that treatments designed to affect brain activation can help CRPS.[30] This subject will be returned to in Chapter 8.

Box 5.8 Possible mechanisms of sympathetic-afferent coupling[22,23,31]

The following hypothetical models are based on animal experiments. Some, but by no means all, are confirmed by observations in humans.

If a nerve is constricted or damaged, the blood vessels and surviving nerves may develop an increased response to catecholamines. This is likely to be due to the increased production (also called expression) of adrenoreceptors in the vessels and axons, creating the false impression that the sympathetic nervous system is overactive.

The vascular receptor changes can be seen as a functional adaptation of the tissues: the increase in receptors may compensate for the reduction in noradrenaline. The effect of the sympathetic denervation on the regulation of local circulation is therefore kept to a minimum. This process can be compared with the upregulation of axonal sodium channels after denervation, which is a functional adaptation in response to a reduction in neurotrophic factor from the periphery (see Ch. 3). Whether this increased expression of adrenoreceptors plays a role in patients with CRPS is not clear, because many do not have a history of overt nerve damage. However, biopsies of the skin of some patients do reveal an increased adrenoreceptor population.

An additional mechanism associated with experimental nerve damage is the growth of sympathetic terminals into the dorsal root ganglion (Fig. 5.9). These sympathetic nerve endings surround the cell bodies of damaged axons. However, because they target thick myelinated nerves and not the nerves usually associated with nociception, it is not clear whether this change is associated with the production of pain.[32]

It is very likely that the early stage of CRPS Type 1 is associated with inflammation. The characteristic swelling, redness and pain are also typical of the inflammatory process. The role of the sympathetic nervous system on the inflammation is not certain. It is possible that noradrenaline does not affect the sensory nerves directly, but by stimulating the release of prostaglandins which in turn sensitize the nerve endings (see Ch. 2).

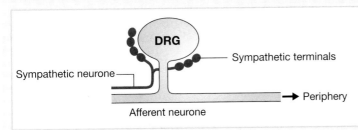

Fig. 5.9 Sympathetic basket formation in the dorsal root ganglion (after [31]). Sympathetic terminals form around the dorsal root ganglion DRG of an afferent neurone.

PSYCHOLOGY AND CRPS

It is not uncommon for conditions of unknown aetiology to be labelled as psychogenic in nature (see Ch. 6) and CRPS is no exception. How exactly psychological processes can create or exacerbate the manifestations of this condition is far from clear.[33] It is hardly surprising that a condition characterized by persistent, bizarre and unpredictable pain that is refractory to treatment, has an effect on the patient's behaviour and wellbeing. Furthermore, sympathetic function is closely linked to anxiety and stress, so it is difficult if not impossible to determine whether psychological changes precipitate sympathetic dysfunction or are caused by it.

A study comparing 25 CRPS Type 1 patients with 44 patients with back pain and 21 with peripheral neuropathy, found no significant differences between groups in terms of reporting of symptoms, illness behaviour and distress.[34] History of childhood abuse and trauma were similar for all groups. Evidence reviewed by Covington also found no evidence of CRPS as a psychogenic condition.[35] However, it is acknowledged that a patient's response to pain may determine the progression of the syndrome. A fear of pain and its implications can easily lead to disuse. As mentioned, demineralization of the bones does occur in CRPS sufferers and may be the result of lack of use and immobilization.

Clinicians are advised to leave the rational diagnosis and treatment of psychological issues to trained professionals (see Ch. 6). The next chapter contains advice regarding referral to a clinical psychologist. However, gaining the patient's confidence, carrying out a thorough examination, giving a rational and understandable explanation and applying the correct treatment are equally important.

SUBJECTIVE EXAMINATION OF CRPS TYPE 1 (After [36,37])

- The symptoms develop after some form of trauma and/or immobilization, usually in the periphery (Table 5.2). It is most commonly one-sided and tends to develop within 4 weeks.
- CRPS is a pain syndrome, so it can only be diagnosed if pain-related changes are present. The pain may be present without any provocation and is often described as burning and deep. The patient may guard the affected limb.
- There are often changes associated with alterations in circulation and sweat production, although they may not be present consistently, if at all. The affected limb may be swollen and can be either red and warm or pale, blue and cold.
- After a while, trophic changes may manifest in the form of altered hair growth, changes in appearance of the nails and poor skin quality.
- The patient may report tremors and loss of strength and endurance of the muscles. It is not clear whether these motor changes are caused by the condition, or whether they are the result of pain.

OBJECTIVE EXAMINATION OF CRPS TYPE 1 (After [36,37])

- There may be allodynia or hyperalgesia, which may be provoked by touch, but also by, for instance, stretch of ligaments or capsule or by thermal stimuli. It is up to the clinician to decide whether these signs are to be expected at that stage of the pathology, or whether they are exaggerated. The sensory changes do not conform to the anatomical boundaries of either the tissues involved or the innervating nerves.
- Oedema may be assessed by measurement of the circumference of the affected limb.
- Objective assessment of vasomotor and sudomotor changes may require specialist equipment and laboratory, but can also be judged clinically. Discoloration, temperature changes and changes in sweatiness can be seen and palpated, and must always be compared with the unaffected side.
- Equipment for the measurement of strength including grip is commonly available in physiotherapy and occupational therapy departments. Private practitioners may wish to invest in some measuring equipment to aid objective assessment.

- Trophic changes can only be observed. The use of photography with the patient's written permission is recommended.
- Demineralization of the bones may be apparent on X-rays. Whether this is due to lack of use and immobilization or the pathological mechanism itself is not certain.
- The diagnostic criteria of CRPS Type 1 can be summed up as follows:

1. History of pain
   + allodynia, hyperalgesia or hyperaesthesia
   + two signs from the following list:
   - Oedema
   - Changes in colour and temperature
   - Changes in sweat production
   - Trophic changes (altered hair growth, skin changes, quality of movement and end feel of passive joint movement, nail changes)
   - Impaired motor function.
2. Characteristics of spontaneous pain
   Some clinicians use a classification based on hypothetical successive stages of the syndrome, but this model has been drawn into question[36,38] (Box 5.9).

Exclusion criteria

The diagnosis of CRPS Type 1 relies on the presence of a cluster of symptoms, rather than on well-defined criteria. The exact symptom cluster varies per patient, and agreement between clinicians is poor.[39] A number of the manifestations can be part of other conditions and can be expected in the early stages following trauma (including surgery). It is therefore easy to diagnose CRPS inappropriately and not treat the actual condition responsible for the symptoms.

CRPS Type 1 can therefore only be diagnosed if all potential physical and psychological causes of the condition have been ruled out. This includes frank nerve damage, the manifestation of which is almost identical, but which is classed as CRPS Type 2.

TREATMENT OF CRPS

Many treatment approaches have been tried in an attempt to control CRPS, but there is almost no reliable evidence of genuine efficacy.[42,43]

There is a general agreement in the literature that lack of use and movement of the affected limb is likely to play a role, which makes physical therapy an essential treatment component by default. It is also generally assumed that it is best to prevent the condition from developing while it is still in its early stages, so early mobilization and exercise can be vital following injury, surgery or removal of a plaster cast.

Box 5.9 Is the three-stage model of CRPS realistic?

Traditionally, the development of CRPS Type 1 has been described in terms of three stages.[40-42] The exact description of these stages varies slightly, but is broadly summarized in Box 5.10. This model has been in widespread use for many years, but recent evidence has drawn its validity into question.[38] In a clinical trial, over 100 patients were matched with a CRPS stage based on clinical manifestations. The assessor was unaware of the history of the symptoms. Comparison of the results with the time course of the symptoms was negative, i.e. there was no correlation between the manifestation of the condition and its duration. However, although the sequential progression of CRPS was not confirmed, three subtypes could be distinguished:

- Mainly vasomotor/trophic changes and motor changes such as weakness and tremor.
- Highest proportion of patients with pain and sensory abnormalities such as allodynia and hyperalgesia. Fewer vasomotor changes than any other group.
- Highest level changes of all groups in terms of pain/sensation, vasomotor activity, sudomotor activity/oedema, and motor activity/trophic status. This group displays all characteristics associated with 'classic RSD'.
- It is yet to be determined whether these subtypes represent different manifestations of the same syndrome, or whether there are three distinct underlying pathologies with similarities in their manifestations.

Stage I The acute or hyperaemic stage

Spontaneous pain/ache/burning
+ hyperpathia/allodynia
± hypoaesthesia/hyperaesthesia
± warmth, dryness and redness of skin.

Stage II The dystrophic or ischemic stage

Radiation of spontaneous pain
+ increased hyperpathia/allodynia
+ cold, cyanotic and sweaty skin
+ decreased hair growth
+ nails cracked, grooved and ridged
+ spreading oedema
+ muscle wasting
+ development of capsular thickening and osteoporosis.

Stage III The atrophic stage, 6–12 months after the initiating event

Pain, hyperpathia and allodynia may reduce
+ decreased blood flow and skin temperature
+ increased/decreased sweating
+ irreversible trophic changes in skin, subcutaneous tissues, muscles and joints.

CONCLUSION

Ongoing pain, psychological distress and regulation of the sympathetic and endocrine systems are inextricably linked. While symptomatic treatment of the pain may result in resolution of the other factors, this is by no means certain. In fact, failure to address HPA function may render any musculoskeletal intervention useless. Some methods of addressing this function have been discussed in this chapter. The psychological factors that play a role in pain and distress are the topic of the following chapter.

One treatment that has been shown to be effective in a long-term study is the 'stress loading' or 'scrub-and-carry' regime for the upper limb.[44] The scrub element of the regime is designed to provide compression. It involves scrubbing the floor whilst leaning on the affected arm for several minutes. The carry portion involves carrying a weight for a few minutes. Over the weeks, time and weight are increased.

Traditionally, therapists have been advised to be vigorous in their approach to CRPS: no pain, no gain. However, there is no evidence for the efficacy of this type of treatment. In fact, it is more likely that the pain and distress created by rough treatment heightens the activity of the sympathetic nervous system, which is potentially involved in creating the symptoms. Treatments that create extreme pain are also likely to discourage the patient from using the affected limb. It is therefore important to encourage use and exercise, along with realistic explanation and reassurance. Mobilization of the joints may be beneficial, but should not exceed the patient's tolerance. Patients who are extremely fearful may benefit from a cognitive-behavioural approach.

Additional treatments may be aimed at the control of swelling in the form of massage, heat and/or cold and constant or intermittent compression. Pain relief may be obtained from the application of gentle manual techniques, acupuncture and various forms of electrotherapy. Because of the lack of evidence, each treatment has to be judged on its merit for the individual.

A recent study describes success with a treatment using movement imagery as a way of addressing cortical function in patients with CRPS.[30] This opens the door for a new approach, akin to treatment used to regain function after stroke. This will be explored in Chapter 8.

If symptoms progress despite manual therapy, advice and exercise, urgent referral to a pain specialist is recommended. Medical treatment may involve adjuvant medication such as the tricyclic drugs or anticonvulsants discussed in Chapter 3. Other approaches involve temporary blockade of the sympathetic nervous system, as reviewed in the medical literature.[45,46] An example is the injection of local anaesthetic into the stellate ganglion or a paravertebral ganglion. The intravenous regional sympathetic block (IVRS) involves emptying the veins of the affected limb and filling them with guanethidine, a drug that blocks the action of noradrenaline. Although statistically the benefits are very limited, some patients make dramatic progress following sympathetic blockade.

The invasive approaches to CRPS are often unpleasant for the patient. Whilst a quickly deteriorating clinical presentation may warrant such an approach, often patients are best served by the appropriate application of physical therapy and guidance.

References

[1] Guyton A, Hall J. Textbook of medical physiology. Philadelphia: WB Saunders 2000

[2] Jänig W. The puzzle of 'Reflex Sympathetic Dystrophy': mechanisms, hypotheses, open questions. In: Jänig W, Stanton-Hicks M, eds. Reflex sympathetic dystrophy: a reappraisal. Seattle: IASP Press, 1996: 1–24

[3] Baron R, Blumberg H, Jänig W. Clinical characteristics of patients with Complex Regional Pain Syndrome in Germany with special emphasis on vasomotor function. In: Jänig W, Stanton-Hicks M, eds. Reflex sympathetic dystrophy: a reappraisal. Seattle: IASP Press, 1996: 25–48

[4] Selye's General Adaptation Syndrome. Available online: http://brain.mhri.edu.au/gap.html 29-11-2003

[5] Hans Selye. Understanding stress 1907–1982. Available online: http://collections.ic.gc.ca/heirloom_series/volume4/222-223.htm 29-11-2003

[6] Youngson R. Hans Selye and the effects of stress. Scientific blunders. London: Constable and Robinson 1998: 230–239

[7] Smelik P. De biologie van stress. Hart bulletin 1982; 13:3–9

[8] de Morree J. Dynamiek van het menselijk bindweefsel. Functie, beschadiging en herstel. Utrecht: Bohn, Scheltema and Holkema, 1989

[9] Melzack R. From the gate to the neuromatrix. Pain 1999; (Supplement 6): S121–S126

[10] Brading A. The autonomic nervous system. Oxford: Blackwell Science, 1999

[11] Iversen S, Iversen L, Saper C. The autonomic nervous system and the hypothalamus. In: Kandel E, Schwartz J, Jessell T, eds. Principles of neural science. New York: McGraw-Hill, 2000: 960–981

[12] Jänig W. Neurologische grondslagen. In: Piët J, Sachs J, Sachs-Piët I, eds. Bindweefselmassage. Lochem: De Tijdstroom, 1989: 22–61

[13] Sato A, Schmidt R. Somatosympathetic reflexes: afferent fibers, central pathways, discharge characteristics. Physiological Reviews 1973; 53(4):16–947

[14] Sato A, Schmidt R. The modulation of visceral functions by somatic afferent activity. Japanese Journal of Physiology 1987; 37:1–17

[15] Piët J, Sachs J, Sachs-Piët I. Bindweefselmassage, 4th edn. Lochem: De Tijdstroom, 1989

[16] Mann F. Reinventing acupuncture. A new concept of ancient medicine, 2nd edn. Oxford: Butterworth Heinemann, 2000

[17] Mayer E, Gebhart G. Basic and clinical aspects of visceral hyperalgesia. Gastroenterology 1994; 107:271–293

[18] Bernstein C, Niazi N, Robert M, Mertz H, Kodner A, Munakata J, et al. Rectal afferent function in patients with inflammatory and functional intestinal disorders. Pain 1996; 66:151–161

[19] Bernards A. Fysiologie en pathofysiology van nocisensoriek. In: van Zutphen H, van Sambeek H, Oostendorp R, van Rens P, Bernards A, eds. Nederlands leerboek der fysische therapie in engere zin – Deel 1. Utrecht: Bunge, 1991

[20] Rothschild B. The body remembers. The psychophysiology of trauma and trauma treatment. London: WW Norton, 2000

[21] Levine P, Frederick A. Waking the tiger. Healing trauma. Berkely, California: North Atlantic Books, 1997

[22] Baron R, Levine J, Fields H. Causalgia and Reflex Sympathetic Dystrophy: does the sympathetic nervous system contribute to the generation of pain? Muscle Nerve 1999; 22:678–695

[23] Jänig W, Häbler H. Sympathetic nervous system: contribution to chronic pain. Prog Brain Res 2000; 129:451–468

[24] Abram S. Incidence-hypothesis-epidemiology. In: Stanton-Hicks M, ed. Pain and the sympathetic nervous system. Boston: Kluwer Academic, 1990: 1–16

[25] Weber M, Birklein F, Neundorfer B, Schmelz M. Facilitated neurogenic inflammation in complex regional pain syndrome. Pain 2001; 91(3):51–257

[26] Abram S. Incidence-hypothesis-epidemiology. In: Stanton-Hicks M, ed. Pain and the sympathetic nervous system. Boston: Kluwer, 1990: 1–16

[27] Guo T-Z, Offley S, Boyd E, Jacobs C, Kingery W. Substance P signaling contributes to the vascular and nociceptive abnormalities observed in a tibial fracture rat model of complex regional pain syndrome type I. Pain 2004; 108(1,2):5–107

[28] Rommel O, Gehling M, Dertwinkel R, et al. Hemisensory impairment in patients with complex regional pain syndrome. Pain 1999; 80(1,2):95–101

[29] Juottonen K, Gockel M, Silen T, Hurri H, Hari R, Forss N. Altered central sensorimotor processing in patients with complex regional pain syndrome. Pain 2002; 98(3):15–323

[30] Mosely G. Graded motor imagery is effective for long-standing complex regional pain syndrome: a randomized controlled trial. Pain 2004; 108(1,2):192–198

[31] Baron R. The influence of sympathetic nerve activity and catecholamines on primary afferent neurons. IASP Newsletter 1998 (May/June)

[32] Ramer M, Thompson S, McMahon S. Causes and consequences of sympathetic basket formation in dorsal root ganglia. Pain 1999; Supplement 6:111–120

[33] Covington E. Psychological issues in reflex sympathetic dystrophy. In: Stanton-Hicks M, Jänig W, eds. Reflex Sympathetic Dystrophy: a reappraisal. Seattle: IASP Press, 1996: 191–216

[34] Ciccone D, Bandilla E, Wu W. Psychological dysfunction in patients with Reflex Sympathetic Dystrophy. Pain 1997; 71(3):323–333

[35] Covington E. Psychological issues in reflex sympathetic dystrophy. In: Stanton-Hicks M, Jänig W, eds. Reflex Sympathetic Dystrophy: a reappraisal. Seattle: IASP Press, 1996: 191–216

[36] Wilson P, Low P, Bedder M, Covington E, Rauck R. Diagnostic algorithm for Complex Regional Pain Syndromes. In: Stanton-Hicks M, Jänig W, eds. Reflex Sympathetic Dystrophy: a reappraisal. Seattle: IASP Press, 1996: 93–106

[37] Jänig W, Baron R. The role of the sympathetic nervous system in neuropathic pain: clinical observations and animal models. In: Hansson P, Fields H, Hill R, Marchetti P, eds. Neuropathic pain: pathophysiology and treatment. Seattle: IASP Press, 2002: 125–149

[38] Bruehl S, Harden R, Galer B, Saltz S, Backonja M, Stanton-Hicks M. Complex regional pain syndrome: are there distinct subtypes and sequential stages of the syndrome? Pain 2002; 95(1–2):19–124

[39] van de Vusse A, Stomp-van den Berg S, de Vet H, Weber W. Interobserver reliability of diagnosis in patients with complex regional pain syndrome. Eur J Pain 2003; 7(3):59–265

[40] Wilson P. Sympathetically maintained pain: diagnosis, measurement, and efficacy of treatment. In: Stanton-Hicks M, ed. Pain and the sympathetic nervous system. Boston: Kluwer, 1990: 91–123

[41] Complex Regional Pain Syndrome. Lecture handout conference British Association of Hand Therapists, Edinburgh: 2000

[42] Wright A. Neuropathic pain. In: Strong J, Unruh A, Wright A, Baxter G, eds. Pain. A textbook for therapists. Edinburgh: Churchill Livingstone, 2002: 351–377

[43] Bengtson K. Physical modalities for complex regional pain syndrome. Hand Clinics 1997; 13(3):43–454

[44] Watson H, Carlson L. Treatment of reflex sympathetic dystrophy of the hand with an active 'stress loading' program. J Hand Surg 1987; 12A(2 Pt 1):779–785

[45] Mackin G. Medical and pharmacological management of upper extremity neuropathic pain syndromes. Journal of Hand Therapy 1997; 10:96–109

[46] Arlet J, Mazieres B. Medical treatment of Reflex Sympathetic Dystrophy. Hand Clinics 1997; 13(3):77–483.

[47] Barker R, Barasi S, Neal M. Neuroscience at a glance. Oxford: Blackwell Science, 2000

[48] van Cranenburgh B. Neurowetenschappen – een overzicht. Maarssen: Elsevier/De Tijdstroom, 1999

[49] Piët J, Sachs J, Sachs-Piët I. Bindweefselmassage, 4th edn. Lochem: De Tijdstroom, 1989

[50] van Dixhoorn J, Duivenoorden H. Efficacy of Nijmegen questionnaire in recognition of the hyperventilation syndrome. J Psychosocial Res 1985; 29(2):99–206.51.

[51] Wilson P. Sympathetically maintained pain: diagnosis, measurement, and efficacy of treatment. In: Stanton-Hicks M, ed. Pain and the sympathetic nervous system. Boston: Kluwer Academic, 1990: 91–123

chronic pain, as popular theorists have emphasized that pain is a psychological as well as a physical experience.[5]

The amount and quality of pain felt is not determined simply by the degree of bodily damage but influenced by previous experiences, learning, memory, understanding, degree of control, cultural background, mood, fears and expectations. What we now know is that the pain signalling system is not a hard-wired structure but is dynamic and plastic; descending pathways in the central nervous system represent the individual's state of mind – memories, experience, fears, expectations and mood. These modulate transmission from the first synapse onwards.[1] In the transition from acute to chronic pain, it has been found that psychological factors have more predictive power than biomedical or biomechanical variables, with respect to disability.[6,7] Addressing these factors at an early stage in treatment can lead to significantly improved outcomes.

THE TRANSITION FROM ACUTE TO CHRONIC PAIN

The *Yellow Flags* approach was first developed as a systematic way to help primary care treatment providers involved in low back care to identify and quantify the psychosocial factors which contributed to long-term disability. The aim was to provide suggestions for management, which would help prevent the development of long-term problems.[8,9]

Kendall[6] identified that psychosocial factors have the potential to influence an acute musculoskeletal pain problem at three distinct phases:

- The onset of pain
- The seeking and receiving of health care and income support
- The development of chronic pain-related disability and work loss.

They suggested that all patients should receive an assessment 2–4 weeks from initial consultation if they are still consulting medical professionals and unable to return to work.

Some patients will require a surgical intervention; at this stage a psychosocial assessment may be important. It has been found that patients with long-standing psychological problems tend to fare poorly in response to spine surgery.[10] Studies of spine surgery outcomes demonstrate that satisfactory relief of pain is achieved anywhere between 16% and 95% of the time in lumber spine fusions[11] with more consistent results achieved in less invasive procedures such as laminectomy and discectomy.[12] The outcome of physical treatments has also been found to be affected by personality[13] and the experience of physical, sexual or emotional abuse.[14] Schofferman et al found that patients who reported at least three types of childhood abuse (sexual, physical, emotional or parental substance abuse or abandonment) had an 85% failure rate with spine surgery compared with a 5% failure rate among patients who reported no such trauma. A growing body of research has demonstrated over the past two decades that psychosocial factors contribute to the variability in spine surgery outcome.[15] Underpinning this research is the basic assumption that pain/disability is a complex phenomenon that consists of a number of factors, each of which can contribute to the interpretation of pain as nociception.[15]

It is not appropriate for a Clinical Psychologist to screen all patients for spine surgery; those spinal disorders that are associated with high surgical success rates mean there is little additional advantage in screening.[16] However, with prolonged pain and emotional distress, adverse and possibly self-perpetuating psychological and social changes may significantly decrease the impact of disc surgery.[17] For patients who are to undergo invasive procedures such as spine surgery, pre-surgical psychological interventions can improve outcome in various ways. These include reducing stress levels, improving motivation, enlisting family support and providing realistic expectations. The development of an individualized treatment plan can improve outcome or provide an alternative to patients for whom surgery has a poor prognosis. Post-surgery, psychological input can assist with patient adjustment and recovery throughout the rehabilitation process.[18]

Pincus et al[19] reiterated that there is good evidence to support the role of psychological risk factors at early stages of low back pain in the development of long-term disability. They also highlighted that there are evidence-based theories and models that provide directions for future interventions. Increasingly research is pointing to the need to assess psychosocial factors at an earlier stage than currently occurs.

PSYCHOSOCIAL ASSESSMENT

Patients may welcome the news that a psychosocial assessment can not establish the relative contributions of organic and psychological factors (nor can any other method, as the underlying model is erroneous). Nor can it establish 'cause and effect' relationships between psychological problems and pain.[20] However, it can help to broaden understanding of the pain problem, and clarify many of the 'vicious circles' that people with chronic pain often fall into; making more explicit the links between their thoughts, physiological responses and behaviour. The assessment may include the administration of standardized questionnaires (see Box 6.1). These questionnaires can also be useful in outcomes based research and evidence-based medicine, and are essential in securing additional funding and demonstrating the efficacy of treatments. For a comprehensive overview of assessment the reader is directed to [21].

The assessment of pain is often a multidisciplinary enterprise, which involves not just quantifying pain per se, but exploring the nature of the pain experience, and what significance the individual assigns to that experience.[5] The multiple components of the pain experience include the following.

- The physiological component, which is concerned primarily with the organic aetiology of the pain.

Box 6.1 Understanding standardized questionnaires

There is a plethora of questionnaires which have been developed to provide a snapshot of some aspect of health, thinking or behaviour. These tests can vary enormously in what they are able to realistically tell us, and are no substitute for a good clinical assessment. However, they can be useful for knowing when to refer on, and good for audit purposes when administered pre- and post-intervention. The choice of questionnaire should be done with care, to ensure that the rest is reliable and valid.

Within psychometrics, two of the most important aspects of a test are its reliability and its validity. *Reliability* is the estimate of the accuracy of a questionnaire. Respondents should obtain a similar score on different occasions providing that they have not changed in a way that would impact on their responses. There are several ways of measuring this. *Test–re-test reliability* involves giving the questionnaire on two occasions and correlating the scores. *Parallel forms* entails constructing two equivalent forms of same questionnaire and giving both to the same people to correlate the scores. *Split-half reliability* involves dividing the questionnaire into two halves and correlating scores to produce an estimate of reliability for the whole questionnaire. *Validity* is the extent to which a questionnaire measures what it is intended to measure. There are several types of validity, namely face validity, content validity, criterion related validity and predictive validity. For any test the reliability and validity must be quoted so the user knows the expected level of error and for whom the questionnaire is intended. Standardization involves obtaining information on the test scores from the general population and generating rules to enable a raw score to have meaning when comparisons are made.[22]

- The sensory component as related to how the pain actually feels to the individual who has it, such as the intensity, location, and quality of the pain.
- The affective component, which is how the pain impacts on mood, outlook, sense of well-being and other emotional states such as fear.
- The cognitive component, which is the way in which the pain influences a person's thought processes or their self-concept. Aspects of this dimension include the meaning of pain, attitudes and beliefs the individual has about their experience of pain, coping skills and strategies.
- The behavioural component, which assesses the behaviours that may be termed pain-related. Behaviours are sometimes performed to decrease the severity of pain, although others are actually indicators of the presence of pain. Many behaviours will increase as the severity of pain increases, and decrease when it lessens. Aspects of the behavioural component include physical activity, medications and treatment interventions.
- Sociocultural dimension of pain. This dimension comprises a broad range of ethnocultural, demographic, spiritual, social, and other factors related to an individual' perception of and response to pain.[23]

A clinical assessment forms the basis of this information gathering, but some standardized questionnaires can supplement this information and also provide useful baselines for audit purposes.

The assessment of the physiological and sensory aspects of pain is covered in several chapters of this book, but some standardized questionnaires concerned with this enterprise can be found on the British Pain Society Website http://www.painsociety.org/pain_scales.html. These are available in a number of different languages.

The discussion below covers the assessment of the other components of pain.

Affective components of pain

Traditional dualistic thinking proposed that the absence of an identified cause for pain was 'repressed' depression.[25] Although there is now ample evidence to refute this model (e.g. [24]), depression can be a consequence of pain, and can also pre-exist pain. Obtaining a measure of depression can aid in tailoring an individual treatment plan. A further discussion on depression is presented later in this chapter.

Physical therapists often worry about discussing mental health issues with patients. However, asking the patient about symptoms of depression or anxiety can communicate hope, in that the patients' symptoms are frequent and understandable. It also communicates that the reality of their problems is being taken seriously. Talking about a 'lowering of spirits' or 'low mood' can be useful;[26] the use of these sort of phrases making it clear that it is not all in the head, but that pain affects mood and vice versa.

There are numerous screening tools available to aid in the detection of depression, but caution needs to be taken in administering these as they are intended to supplement assessment by a clinician trained in mental health. However, Aroll et al[27] suggested that two questions have reasonable sensitivity and specificity to detect depression in a primary care setting. These are:

- 'During the past month, have you often been bothered by feeling down, depressed or hopeless?'
- 'During the past month, have you often been bothered by little interest or pleasure in doing things?'

Although it would be prudent to not assume that a person is depressed on the basis of just two questions, they may help in the decision to refer on to a clinical psychologist or other mental health professional.

Three instruments, the Beck Depression Inventory (BDI),[28] the Distress and Risk Assessment Scale (DRAM)[29] and The Hospital Anxiety and Depression Scale (HAD)[30] were developed specifically to identify mood changes. None of the instruments take more than 5 minutes to administer, and most can be done in 2 or 3 minutes.

The *Beck Depression Inventory 1996 (BDI–II)* consists of 21 questions, each rated for intensity on a scale of 0–3, reflecting attitudes often displayed by depressed people. In each, zero represents normality and 3 represents severe disturbance. It can not be used to diagnose depression in the absence of a diagnosis, but it is a measure of severity once the diagnosis has been made.[31] Unfortunately, chronic pain patients often obtain high scores on somatic factors (such as poor sleep) and low scores on self-denigratory cognitive items (i.e. blaming cognitions), unlike the uni-dimensional structure characteristic of depressed populations in which affective and cognitive items dominate.[32] This means that a high score may not be a true reflection of depression, but instead reflect the functional changes that accompany chronic pain.

The *Distress and Risk Assessment Method (DRAM)*[29] is widely used across the UK. This test was specifically developed to identify distress in those with chronic back pain, and alert clinicians to the need for a more comprehensive assessment, after recognition that psychosocial factors affect the outcome of spine surgery and impact on the level of disability. Patients are classified into those showing no psychological distress, those at risk of developing major psychological overlay and those clearly distressed. The DRAM consists of the Modified Somatic Perceptions Questionnaire (MSPQ), which consists of 22 items to measure heightened somatic awareness, and the Modified Zung (MZ), which is a 23-item self-report measure of depression. Somatic awareness is expanded upon later in this chapter, but can be thought of as an increased focus on the body and selective attention to certain body sensations, which lowers the threshold for perceiving sensations, and increases the subjective intensity of these events.

Another widely used questionnaire to measure mood is the *Hospital Anxiety and Depression Scale (HAD)*. Although this was designed for use on hospital populations, research is suggesting that depression in chronic pain is qualitatively different in terms of cognitive content from classical depression, and more discriminating measures should be used. Chronic pain patients can obtain a clinically significant score on most depression measures by checking items measuring sleep disturbance, fatigue, reduced activity etc. There is a need for measures which account for the somatic aspects of pain.[32] A more comprehensive discussion of depression in chronic pain is provided later in this chapter.

Cognitive aspects of pain

The meaning of the pain to the individual is important. In the Western world pain has typically been linked with punishment, torture and damnation.[33] Communicating the meaning of the pain is highly important and may necessitate the use of creative techniques.[34]

The way a person thinks about their pain and the behaviours they engage in will have a significant impact on the ability to effectively cope with pain. *Catastrophic thoughts* and *coping strategies* affect not only the level of pain, but also the ability to overcome and adjust to pain. Catastrophizing is explained in more detail later in this chapter. The *Pain-Related Self Statements*[35] self-report questionnaire consists of 18 items to measure catastrophizing (9 items) and active coping (9 items). The *Pain Self-Efficacy Questionnaire*[36] is a 10-item, self-report questionnaire designed to measure how confident the patient feels in coping with their pain. Research has shown that on the *Coping Strategies Questionnaire*,[37] patients who responded well to surgery tended to perceive themselves as having some control over their ability to control and reduce the pain. In terms of external factors, spousal reinforcement[38] is associated with increased pain behaviour, although the precise way in which these factors influence outcome is not known.

Krir[39] identified the importance of helping patients develop more proactive coping strategies, and not engage in avoidance of pain and movement. The Coping Strategies Questionnaire 24[40] can be a clinically quick and useful way of identifying the specific ways in which patients cope.

Pain beliefs and cognitions have been shown to predict functioning in chronic pain patients.[41] The *Pain Beliefs and Perceptions Inventory (PBPI)* is a 16-item scale measuring the extent of agreement or disagreement about certain beliefs about pain. It consists of four scales:

- Mystery: the belief that the pain is mysterious or poorly understood
- Self-blame: the belief that one is responsible for one's pain
- Permanence: the belief that the pain will be a permanent part of one's life
- Constancy: the belief that the pain is and will be a chronic problem.

Behavioural aspects of pain

Pain can not be seen, but is expressed and communicated in immensely varied ways: in shivers; moans; winces; social and physical withdrawal.[34] The function of pain is to demand attention and prioritize escape, recovery, and healing; where others can help achieve these goals, effective communication of pain is required.[42]

In exploring the communication of pain, clinicians have focused on 'pain behaviours' such as guarding, touching, sounds, words, and facial expression, which serve to communicate pain. Waddell and colleagues[43] identified a series of non-organic signs that may appear in low back pain patients. These so termed 'Waddell signs' (WSs) are a group of eight physical findings divided into five categories, the presence of which has been suggested to indicate malingering, secondary gain, hysteria, psychological distress, magnified presentation, abnormal illness behaviour, abnormal pain behaviour, and somatic amplification. However, a recent evidence-based review of the research on WSs which took account of strength and consistency of findings concluded that:

- WSs do not correlate with psychological distress
- WSs do not discriminate organic from non-organic problems
- WSs may represent an organic phenomenon
- WSs are associated with poorer treatment outcome
- WSs are associated with greater pain levels
- WSs are not associated with secondary gain.[44]

Waddell noted that there is a tremendous variation in the individual response to chronic pain according to its context and the meaning to the sufferer, and the relationship between pain, distress and disability is dynamic and multidimensional.[43] In addition, communication is a two-way process, and it is interesting that experience with patients who have pain influences subjective ratings of pain. Prkachin et al[45] found that observers with a positive family history of chronic pain attributed greater pain to the patients than those with a negative family history of chronic pain. Professionals' pain judgements were lower than those of control subjects. It has also been found that people need careful training in assessing pain behaviours and facial pain in particular may not be a reliable way of assessing pain[42]. Thoughts/cognitions also impact on pain behaviours. Research into *self-efficacy* has shown that the more confident a patient feels in terms of coping with their pain, the less they avoid movement and activities over an extended period.[46] Self-efficacy is an important determinant of pain behaviours and disability associated with pain, over and above the effects of pain, distress and personality variables. Consequently, trying to assess 'pain behaviours' without considering the meaning of these behaviours to the individual is highly problematic. What may be more helpful is to measure functional ability. Functional questionnaires such as the *Roland-Morris Disability Questionnaire*[47] are discussed in more depth in Chapter 8.

Sociocultural aspects of pain

In recent years, pain management programmes have recognized the importance of assessing and addressing external factors such as relationships with family members and employers, and the impact of litigation claims.[38,48]

The research by Flor et al[38] has been very useful in highlighting that an over-protective partner/spouse is not helpful for pain patients, as they reinforce the idea of fear of harm or catastrophic thinking. Taking over household tasks is not helpful in the long-term, as it contributes to disuse and depression. Equally, a punitive response from family members is not helpful, as is not being able to discuss the problems associated with having chronic pain. Recent research has shown that plastic changes in the brain occur in response to this conditioned response,[48] and consequently at a physiological level, behavioural changes are mapped.

There are also several issues to do with employment which affect outcome and increasingly pain management programmes are recognizing the importance of including employment related components.[49] These are expanded on later in this chapter.

PSYCHOLOGICAL THERAPY

Many professionals are uncertain about the role of a clinical psychologist. This section aims to provide an overview of the role, which should aid in onward referral.

Clinical psychologists aim to reduce psychological distress and to enhance and promote psychological well-being. They work with people with mental or physical health problems, which might include anxiety and depression, serious and enduring mental illness, adjustment to physical illness, neurological disorders, addictive behaviours, childhood behaviour disorders, personal and family relationships. They work with people throughout the lifespan and with those with learning disabilities.

Within the area of pain management, clinical psychologists have an important role in identifying psychosocial risk factors and helping patients to make choices that will help enhance mental and emotional well-being. Making explicit the links between how a person thinks, and their behaviour and physiology, can enable the patient to gain some control over the 'vicious cycles' that have come to dominate their life. Patients with chronic conditions can have negative or unhelpful ways of thinking; often feeling hopeless or helpless about a situation. Past psychological issues can impact on how people cope with pain, and addressing these through psychological therapy can often help the patient benefit from other physical treatments. In the majority of cases the clinical psychologist is an integral part of the multidisciplinary pain team, as the multidimensional nature of pain often means the complexity needs to be addressed from a number of angles.

Clinical psychologists work from a broad theoretical base to formulate a clinical approach to people's problems. This 'formulation' is an alternative to diagnosis, and may be revised using a different theoretical perspective as the therapy progresses and more information comes to light. Psychologists also work at different levels to try to maximize the application of psychological ideas. Their role includes working directly with individuals and groups of patients, teaching, supervision of other professionals, teamwork and research and audit. Clinical psychologists also have skills to meet the challenges of the modern NHS, with its commitment to flexibility and the need to improve service delivery and outcome. They are trained to reflect on practice and consider alternative ways of meeting patients needs, to improve health and reduce health inequalities. The British Psychological Society is the Professional body for Psychologists; more information about this can be found at: www.bps.org.uk

A patient's first appointment with the clinical psychologist can seem scary, associated with psychiatric labels and 'all in the mind' statements, which mark the end of the pain being taken seriously by doctors. Some don't even attend the initial meeting and many patients spend the first minutes emphasizing their sanity and the reality of their pain. Physical therapists and other health professionals can play a valuable role in preparing people for a psychological assessment, by explaining the multidimensional nature of chronic pain and helping the patient to understand that the clinical psychologist is one part of treating a complex problem.

Clinical psychologists draw from a number of theoretical frameworks to formulate and work with a presenting problem.[50] Cognitive-behavioural therapy dominates the pain field and evidence based practice; its structured format lending itself to the scrutiny of randomized controlled trials. Beck[51] has argued that cognitive therapy is *the* integrative therapy although others would disagree. It would be impossible to provide an overview of all theoretical models here, but an outline of the main approaches is provided.

COGNITIVE-BEHAVIOUR THERAPY

Cognitive-behaviour therapy (CBT) aims to reduce the potency of negative (catastrophic) thoughts, and use behavioural principles to tackle avoided movements and activities in a graded way. It was developed by Aaron Beck.[52]

Cognitive-behavioural approaches are characterized by being focused in the present, being time-limited and structured, and the therapist plays an active role in the therapy. Patients are encouraged to identify and monitor the impact of negative (catastrophic) thinking on their movements, mood, physiology and behaviour (Fig. 6.1).

Cognitive-behavioural treatment is a collaborative approach that aims to develop problem solving skills, promote acceptance and counter the helplessness and withdrawal that can accompany more passive treatment modalities. Patients are encouraged to test out their appraisals, expectations and beliefs through 'behavioural experiments', and start to challenge these in a graded way. Through focusing on improving coping skills and developing a better quality of life, reliance on health care is often reduced and many patients resume household activites or return to employment.[53]

Catastrophic thinking, or worry can be defined as:

'A chain of thoughts and images, negatively affect laden and relatively uncontrollable. The worry process represents an attempt to engage in mental problem solving on an issue whose outcome is uncertain but contains the possibility of one or more negative outcomes' ([55], p. 10).

Making negative interpretations of events has been observed to occur in the thoughts of people suffering from anxiety.[52] Often chronic pain patients catastrophize about the meaning of their pain and worry about the future.[56] Their cognitions centre on the worst possible outcome and this leads them to avoid doing anything 'dangerous' in terms of physical activity. This fear is associated with increased psychophysiological reactivity (as discussed in Ch. 5), when the individual is faced with situations they appraise as 'dangerous' and which make physical activity more dangerous.[2] Pain is maintained through hypervigilance towards painful sensations and subsequent avoidance. The increasing focus on the body and selective attention to certain body sensations lowers the threshold for perceiving sensations and increases the subjective intensity of these events. The patients can develop safety behaviours aimed at preventing feared catastrophes and get into unhelpful patterns of thinking and behaviour.[57] Longstanding avoidance and physical inactivity has a detrimental impact on the musculoskeletal and cardiovascular systems, leading to 'disuse syndrome'.[58] Avoidance also leads to withdrawal from pleasurable activities, which leads to mood disturbance such as irritability, depression and frustration. Hasenbring et al[7] found that among the pain-related cognitions, catastrophizing and fear-avoidance-beliefs had the most empirical support for predicting long-term disability and Crombez et al[59] found that pain related fear may be more disabling than pain itself.

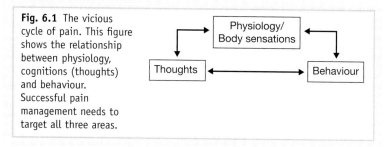

Fig. 6.1 The vicious cycle of pain. This figure shows the relationship between physiology, cognitions (thoughts) and behaviour. Successful pain management needs to target all three areas.

Cognitive-behavioural models contend that fear of pain and appraisals of harm affect the individual's behaviour and impact on chronicity.[2] This is termed fear avoidance (Fig. 6.2). Negative appraisals about pain and its consequences, such as catastrophic thinking (Box 6.2), are thought of as a precursor of pain related fear.[54]

Eccleston[56] identified the subjective impact of chronic pain. Pain leads people to increasingly focus on their bodies, and 'normal' sensation becomes lost as the pain takes over. Pain increasingly interrupts your day, which in turn reduces the amount of time you concentrate on other things. This increases the threat of pain. Catastrophic thoughts are perceived as a threat (fear of pain/damage), which triggers the fight/flight response. The patient shows symptoms of autonomic hyperactivity such as muscle tension, dizziness, a dry mouth, sweating, racing thoughts, churning stomach, feelings of nausea and an increased heart rate. This activation of the autonomic nervous system is a normal and appropriate response to stress but becomes pathological when it is disproportionate to the severity of the stress, continues after the stressor has gone, or occurs in the absence of any external stressor.[60] Figure 6.3 shows the cognitive model of panic (adapted from Clark[61]).

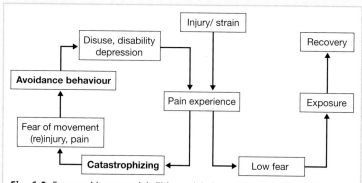

Fig. 6.2 Fear avoidance model. This model shows catastrophic thinking can contribute to a fear of particular movements, and in the longer-term lead to disuse, disability and depression. Reprinted from Pain 62, Fear of movement/(re)injury in chronic low back pain and its relation to behavioural performance, 363–372, 1995, with permission from the *International Association for the Study of Pain*.

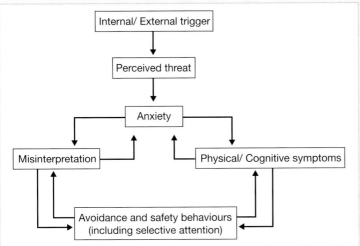

Fig. 6.3 Cognitive model of panic. This figure highlights how an internal (e.g. pain) or external (e.g. seeing someone in a wheelchair) can lead to the perception of a threat. This leads to physiological changes within the body, as well as changes in thinking, which impact on behaviour. Erroneous beliefs about the meaning of these symptoms maintain the perception of threat.

One of the difficulties for the chronic pain patient is that the pain constitutes a problem without an acceptable solution. In the face of a persistent and inescapable source of threat, the patient often becomes chronically vigilant for somatic changes, providing the ideal environment for chronic worry to flourish.[56] Dehghani et al[62] published research, which suggested that patients with chronic pain problems selectively attend to sensory aspects of pain. However, selective attention appears to depend upon the nature of pain stimuli. For those who are highly fearful of pain they may not only selectively attend to pain-related information but have difficulty disengaging from those stimuli.

Eccleston et al[56] found that worries about pain typically fell into one of four categories:

- Pain experience (e.g. 'this pain just keeps hurting')
- Disability (e.g. 'I can't do the ironing')
- Medical uncertainty (e.g. 'is this is a new pain')
- Negative affect (e.g. 'I'm useless').

The average patient worried once a day, for a period of 20 minutes and the worry was likely to be triggered by an increase in pain. Compared with non-pain-related worries, the worry was more difficult to dismiss, more distracting, more attention-grabbing, more intrusive, more distressing and less pleasant. Eccleston's work suggested that worry in chronic pain was not a form of a *Generalized Anxiety Disorder*, but was a normal process that is triggered by the abnormal situation of chronic pain. McCracken and Eccleston found that accept-

The Stroop Task is a test of mental flexibility and vitality. It takes advantage of our ability to read words quicker than we can name colours. The cognitive process involved is called inhibition. Individuals have to read a list of colours, that are themselves presented in different colours such as **Green** written in blue ink. Humans have to invest a lot of effort to suppress the natural instinct to read a word, and the Stroop Task is sensitive to effects of fatigue.

The task of making an appropriate response – when given two conflicting signals – has tentatively been located in a part of the brain called the *anterior cingulate*. This is a region that lies between the right and left halves of the frontal portion of the brain. It is involved in a wide range of thought processes and emotional responses.

You can take the Stroop Task on-line at:

http://www.snre.umich.edu/eplab/demos/st0/stroopdesc.html

ance of chronic pain was associated with less pain, disability, depression and pain-related anxiety, higher daily uptime, and better work status.[63]

Changes in attention have been shown to affect pain, through functional imaging techniques. Derbyshire et al[64] discussed how functional imaging techniques have revealed an extensive central network associated with pain. This network includes the thalamus, insula, prefrontal cortex and anterior cingulate cortex (ACC) as well as the somatosensory cortices. Positron emission tomography (PET) of regional cerebral blood flow (rCBF) has demonstrated activation of the ACC during cognitively challenging tasks such as the Stroop interference task (Box 6.3) and divided attention.

Catastrophic thoughts and the resultant fear can also influence paraspinal muscle function; Watson et al examined the impact of psychological factors in abnormal paraspinal activity in patients with chronic low back pain.[65] They found significant correlations between fear avoidance beliefs, low pain self-efficacy and Flexion Relaxation Ratios (FFRs). Treatment on a pain management programme reduced fear avoidance and improved self-efficacy and FFRs improved.

LEARNING AND AVOIDANCE BEHAVIOUR

Pavlov demonstrated that all mammals can learn behaviours over time. Experiments to demonstrate the principles of classical conditioning showed that a response (i.e. salivation) to the pairing of two stimuli (e.g. food and a tone) can be elicited even if the conditioned stimulus (i.e. the tone) is removed. Ideas from classical conditioning can be usefully applied in the chronic pain field. Over time fear of pain may become associated with an expanding number of situations and activities, which patients then avoid. Health providers themselves may become potent cues for chronic pain patients. A patient who has received painful treatment from a physiotherapist may be conditioned to experience a negative emotional response in the presence of, or even in anticipation of the therapist. This negative response will in turn increase muscle tension and amplify pain.[53] Research has shown that negative responses from spouses can lead to plastic changes in the brain[38] and this is equally applicable to health professionals. It is very important to be aware that your response can influence the patient's behaviour and subjective experience of pain.

As seen from the Vlaeyen model (Fig. 6.2), catastrophic thinking leads to fear of pain and fear of movement, which in turn leads to avoidance. Hasenbring et al[7] researched the correlation between ways of coping and disability. They found that passive coping strategies such as avoidance behaviour was one of the most important predictors. It was also found that patients who tended to suppress or ignore pain in order to finish all activities they started, or who were unable to integrate phases of passive relaxation into the daily routine, displayed a high risk of chronicity of pain 6 months after an acute phase of pain. Physical therapists can play a vital role in helping patients to tackle unhelpful ways of coping and avoidance behaviour at an early stage. It is important to emphasize that any avoidance of an activity is temporary, and that as the recovery process advances, things can change and the patient will be able to do more in time. Even teaching people how to do things (e.g. lifting) may be counter-productive, as it suggests that the pain is conditional and may create pain and anxiety when the patient is unable to carry out the activity in the prescribed manner (e.g. when a restriction in available space does not allow them to lift in a certain way).

'Graded exposure' is the treatment of choice for trying to reduce fear.[66] Similar ideas used in the treatment of simple phobias (such as a fear of spiders) can be used to tackle fear avoidance. A hierarchy of feared activities is constructed with the patient, who is then encouraged to break these down into a hierarchy of components and 'expose' themselves to these in a step-wise fashion. The patient is encouraged to use breathing and relaxation techniques, self-talk and other cognitive strategies to help tackle the anxiety generated by the feared movement.

Van Tulder et al[66] reviewed behavioural treatment for chronic non-specific low back pain and concluded that it was effective, but said that it is not known what type of patients will benefit from which treatments.

DISUSE, DISABILITY AND DEPRESSION

As described by Merskey and Bogduk for the International Association for the Study of Pain,[67] 'Pain is unquestionably a sensation in a part or parts of the body, but it is also always unpleasant and therefore also an emotional experience'.

As pain becomes more chronic, psychological variables play an increasingly dominant role in the maintenance of pain behaviours and suffering. These changes are likely to be due to the constant discomfort, despair and preoccupation with the pain, which comes to dominate these patients' lives. However, as stressed earlier, pain is not caused by depression,[68] but can pre-exist the pain.

Within the general population, depression is the most frequent mental health problem; one study estimated the lifetime prevalence in the community at 17%.[68] People become depressed for many reasons, and can have a variety of presentations.[69] These can include a persistent low mood, loss of interest or pleasure in usual activities, crying, feelings of inadequacy, or guilt; feeling resentful, irritable or angry, sleep and/or appetite disturbance and psychomotor agitation or retardation.[26] No reliable biological markers or valid behavioural tests exist that can help define the exact nature of depression and disentangle issues of comorbid pathologies, or co-occurring syndromes or clusters of symptomatology. Accordingly, diagnostic and classification systems have principally relied upon clinical description and the naming of behavioural signs and symptoms to define the syndrome (e.g. sad mood, sleep difficulties, diminished interest). Recent advances

blame themselves for not being a 'good enough' patient, or puzzles over whether it is 'all in their head' and they are going mad. Explaining to patients at an early stage that chronic pain is often unaccompanied by a straightforward physical cause may help enormously in enabling them to construct a more helpful narrative. Clinical psychologists, through psychological therapy, can help to address unhelpful narratives that are impacting on mood and behaviour.

PSYCHODYNAMIC PSYCHOTHERAPY

There are a huge number of psychodynamic psychotherapies, but some of the central ideas are useful when working with chronic pain patients. The more distressed a client group is, the more unconscious communications are likely to predominate, and lead to the team operating in unhelpful ways. By noticing and reflecting on experiences staff can recognize when they become caught up in 'projective identification' with their clients, and think through more helpful ways of working.[81]

Transference and countertransference are both normal phenomena that may arise during the course of the therapeutic relationship.[82] Transference is the 'transference' of the patients' past feelings, conflicts, and attitudes into present relationships, situations, and circumstances. People develop habits, attitudes and preconceived ideas based on the learning and retention of information from past relationships, which then influence subsequent relationships. Countertransference is the term for the feelings the patient subsequently elicits in the health professional.

Becoming more aware of the feelings elicited with different patients can improve practice. This applies to physical therapists as well. The feelings elicited can help develop a better understanding of the patient and can help the therapist to protect themselves from taking on these feelings too much, so as not to succumb to illness, despair and withdrawal or get so entangled in the clients' feelings as to be unable to work with them. Different patients bring out different emotions, both pleasant and unpleasant. It is not helpful to censor these feelings, and having a flexible self-concept is an important part of being able to accept some of the more difficult feelings that certain patients bring out. Trying to 'walk in the patient's shoes' can help foster acceptance of the patient's current situation. It can be helpful to remember that an interaction with a patient is one event in a change process, which can extend over a long period rather than being the ultimate cure.[83] This perspective is very different from the cure-based medical model.

'*Splitting*' means dividing feelings into different elements (e.g. good and bad) and is often accompanied by *projection*, which means locating feelings in other people. Early in childhood splitting and projection are the main ways of avoiding pain, and as a state of mind can occur throughout life. 'Chronic niceness' can develop when staff split off and deny the negative aspects of caring daily for people who are demonstrating they are in a great deal of pain. There can be a collective fantasy that the staff are nice people who are caring for nice people in pain who are going to be cured of the pain. This can protect staff from facing the fact that many people continue to live with a great deal of pain, which is disturbingly not nice. So that this can be maintained, less nice feelings are split off and displaced outside of the staff group; instead managers can be seen as the 'bad' people. Of course there can be very real organizational pressure from managers, but it can also indicate that the staff have moved towards the paranoid-schizoid position in order to retain staff cohesiveness. Sometimes unpleasant feelings are located in one particular member of the team, who ends up leaving because the levels of feeling become intolerable.[84] Readers may recognize this in their area of practice.

Winnicott[85] introduced the idea of the 'good enough mother' and this can equally apply to those in the helping professions. There will be times when disturbed, angry, frightened and dependent patients may give rise to feelings of hate and other negative emotions; this is usual. In turn other patients may elicit strong positive feelings, but the hospital system often does not encourage staff to be moved by their experiences and staff often keep these to themselves.

SYSTEMIC WORK

In many cases it is important to consider not only the individual with pain, but also their family and friends, as people are interdependent. In psychological therapy, family systems theory places special emphasis upon understanding family process within a broader sociocultural context. Systems work explores relationships (at micro and macro levels) and is sensitized to issues of power and the ways in which structured inequalities shape family process and human relationships. There are many branches of family systems theory, and the interested reader is directed towards The Institute of Family Therapy: http://www.instituteoffamilytherapy.org.uk/.

Some central ideas may be helpful from this perspective; it has been found that those patients whose partners reinforce pain behaviours by 'caring too much' have higher levels of disability.[46,47] Involving the partner and other family members to effect change can be an important part of successful work, and can also be important for physiotherapists. Helping the spouse to understand chronic pain and tackle their own fears about the patient taking graded risks, can be important to prevent homework tasks being stopped. It is imperative that the patient and spouse are treated as a team working to overcome the difficulties of chronic pain, and are not treated in a condescending or punitive way. Involving the spouse in the construction of a graded hierarchy, and encouraging the patient to gradually take back some of the tasks the partner now does is an effective way of structuring work (Box 6.5).

The system outside of the family can also be important to work with. Addressing issues in the wider social arena can be more pressing to the individual, and can have a big impact in a relatively short space of time. This can include working with an individual's employer.

Box 6.5   Case example

DG had been extensively investigated with no underlying pathology found for his chronic back pain. He arrived for his appointment in a wheelchair, and demonstrated a high level of disability. His wife accompanied him and insisted on staying with him at all times, maintaining that she would stay in case he needed anything. When the physiotherapist outlined the exercises, DG's wife expressed her anxiety that this would cause further harm. DG informed the physiotherapist that his GP had told them that he should not be moving at all.

Explaining the nature of chronic pain to DG and his wife was the first step in improving his function. Discussing the meaning of previous tests (e.g. MRI) helped them to start to understand that pain does not always equal damage. They were shown the Vlaeyen model and this was fleshed out with their own particular cognitions and behaviours. DG started doing exercises in his wheelchair, but as his confidence increased he felt able to stand and move on to doing exercises without this aid. Simultaneously, his and his wife's fears were tackled during the session using cognitive-behavioural techniques. It was important to start at a low enough level for DG to feel able to start to move; even one movement is better than none. It was also necessary to address issues related to DG's mother who had also been limiting his function. She was lonely and had found helping DG had renewed her sense of worth. Finding her other activities within the local community helped to take her focus away from DG and stopped her from taking over household tasks.

EMPLOYMENT AND BENEFITS

In recent years pain management programmes have recognized the importance of specifically addressing employment issues.[65] Pain can have a tremendous impact on employment, and often if the job was very physical the person is unable to return to their original job. Although Government initiatives change over time, this section provides a broad introduction to present schemes.

The New Deal initiative developed by the British government provides many schemes to assist people with disabilities. In the UK, all these schemes can be accessed through the help of the local Disability Employment Advisor, who is located at the Job Centre. DEAs conduct an employment assessment, and can provide a range of support, advice, training and information. They can refer for a period of 'Work Preparation', which is an individually tailored programme for disabled people to help them to return to work after a period of sickness or unemployment. They can give information on the 'Job Introduction Scheme', which pays a grant to an employer for the first few weeks of a job, or 'Workstep' which provides supported job opportunities for disabled people facing more complex employment barriers.

There are also 'Access to Work advisers'. Access to Work provides money to buy specialist equipment or support (e.g. someone to communicate for a person with a hearing impairment) for the workplace, and is available to those whose disability is likely to last for 12 months or longer, whether they are in employment or not. The Department for Work and Pensions has more about these schemes at: http://www.dwp.gov.uk/.

A government funded charity 'Employment Opportunities' has local branches across the UK, and provides training, advice and support to people with a disability. They can help with CV writing, identifying suitable employers and monitoring a work placement to ensure that any problems are ironed out at an early stage. Their aim is 'to achieve a society where the full potential of people with disabilities is recognized in every workplace.' Find out more at : http://www.opportunities.org.uk/.

Many people are unsure if they are eligible for disability benefits. The Department for Work and Pensions now has a website (http://www.disabilitybenefits.co.uk/) covering these issues and a national helpline (National Helpline Direct Tel: 08457 123456). The Benefit Enquiry Line (0800 88 22 00) is a confidential telephone service available for people with disabilities, their representatives and their carers.

Disability Living Allowance (DLA) is paid to people if they have needed help for three months because of a severe illness or disability, and are likely to need it for another six months. The benefit is not means tested, so is not dependent on income or savings, but on disability. There is a care component (higher, middle and lower rate) and a mobility component (higher rate and lower rate). Forms are available from local Social Security offices or download a form from: http://www.disabilitybenefits.co.uk/.

Disabled person's tax credit is paid to people who are working more than 16 hours but are at a disadvantage getting a job because of illness or disability. Savings over £16 000 means people are ineligible for the benefit. It is paid to people who have been getting one of the following because of an illness or disability in the last 26 weeks: Short-term Incapacity Benefit paid at a higher rate; Long-term Incapacity Benefit; Severe Disablement Allowance; Disability premium or higher pensioner premium on:

- Income Support
- Minimum Income Guarantee
- Income-based Jobseeker's Allowance
- Housing benefit or Council Tax Benefit.

It is also available to people receiving Disability Living Allowance, Attendance Allowance, Industrial Injuries Disablement Benefit paid with Constant Attendance Allowance or an invalid three-wheeler supplied by the Department for Work and Pensions. More information is available on the helpline: 0845 605 58 58.

Incapacity benefit is paid if statutory sick pay has ended, and the patient has paid National Insurance contributions. Incapacity Benefit can be paid at three different rates: Short-term Incapacity Benefit at the lower rate, Short-term Incapacity Benefit at the higher rate and Long-term Incapacity Benefit if you have been sick for over 52 weeks.

References

[1] Wall P. The science of suffering. London: Weidenfeld and Nicholson, 1999

[2] Vlaeyen JWS, Seelen HAM, Peters M, de Jong P, et al. Fear of movement/(re)injury, avoidance and muscular reactivity in chronic low back pain patients. An experimental investigation. Pain 1999; 82:297–304

[3] Banks SM and Kerns RD. Explaining high rates of depression in chronic pain a stress-diathesis framework. Psychol Bull 1996; 199:95–110

[4] Jensen MC, Kelly AP, Brant-Zawadzki MN. MRI of degenerative disease of the lumbar spine. Magn Reson Q 1994; 10(3)173–190

[5] Melzack R, Wall P. The challenge of pain. London: Penguin; 1988

[6] Kendall, NA. Psychosocial approaches to the prevention of chronic pain: the low back paradigm. B Pr Res Clin Rheum 1999; 13(3):545–554

[7] Hasenbring M, Hallner D, Klasen B. [Psychological mechanisms in the transition from acute to chronic pain: over- or underrated?]German. Schmerz 2001; 15(6):442–447

[8] Watson PJ, Booker CK, Main CJ. Evidence for the role of psychological factors in abnormal paraspinal activity in patients with chronic low back pain. J Musculoskeletal Pain 1997; 5(4):41–56

[9] Gatchel RJ, Polatin PB, Mayer TG. The dominant role of psychosocial risk factors in the development of chronic low back pain disability. Spine 1995; 20(24):2702–2709

[10] Manniche C, Ammussen KH, Vinterberg H, et al. Analysis of pre-operative prognostic factors in first-time surgery for lumbar disc herniation, including Finneson's and modified Spengler's score systems. Dan Med Bull 1994; 41: 110–115

CONCLUSION

The expression of emotions during difficult life events is normal and adaptive. However, pain is an adverse event, and has a major impact on individual and family functioning. Many professionals are concerned about perceptions of stigma associated with mental illness and try to avoid labelling their patients. Others assume that psychological distress and depression are to be expected, and try to work with psychological issues during a routine appointment, not bothering to refer on.[86] However, given the time constraints that are imposed on physiotherapists, the possible lack of a private space to discuss personal issues (private practitioners may be better off in this respect) and in many cases a lack of expertise in dealing with distress, there may be many occasions when referral to a clinical psychologist is appropriate.

This chapter has provided an overview of how clinical psychologists work, which will enable physiotherapists to onwardly refer when appropriate. Where there is uncertainty about a referral, talking it through with your local clinical psychologist can be helpful. It may be possible to obtain supervision on certain psychological issues to enable more rewarding work with a particular patient, and develop knowledge and understanding of how psychosocial issues impact on physiology and movement.

The chapter has highlighted that dualistic thinking is not helpful for either the patient or the professional, and any chronic condition requires multidisciplinary work. This is ideally underpinned by individual patient plans that assess and plan for not only the physiological and sensory aspects of pain, but also the affective, cognitive, behavioural and social aspects.

[11] Turner JAM, Herron L Haselkorn J, et al. Patient outcomes after lumbar spinal fusions. JAMA 1992; 268:907–911

[12] Hoffman RM, Wheeler KJ, Deyo RA. Surgery for herniated lumbar discs: a literature synthesis. J Gen Intern Med 1993; 8:487–496

[13] Long C. The relationship between surgical outcome and MMPI profiles in chronic pain patients. J Clin Psychol 1991; 37:744–749

[14] Schofferman J, Anderson D, Hinds R, et al. Childhood psychological trauma correlates with unsuccessful lumbar spine surgery. Spine1992; 17:138–144

[15] Block AR. Presurgical psychological screening. New Jersey: Lawrence Erlbaum Associates,1996

[16] Carragee EJ. Psychological screening in the surgical treatment of lumbar disc herniation. Clin J Pain 2001; 17(3):215–219

[17] Carragee E. Indications for lumbar microdiscectomy. Instr Course Lect 2002; 51:223–228

[18] Gatchell R. A biopsychosocial overview of pre-treatment screening of patients with pain. Clin J Pain 2001; 17:192–199

[19] Pincus T, Vlaeyen JW, Kendall NA, et al. Cognitive-behavioral therapy and psychosocial factors in low back pain: directions for the future. Spine 2002; 27(5): E133–138

[20] Doleys DM. Psychological assessment for implantable therapies. Pain Digest 2000; (10):16–23

[21] Turk DC, Melzack R, eds. Handbook of pain assessment. London: Guildford Press, 1992

[22] Rust J, Golombok S. Modern psychometrics: the science of psychological assessment. London: Routledge, 1992

[23] Greenwald, HP. Interethnic differences in pain perception. Pain 1991; 44:157–163

[24] Blumer D, Heilbronn M, Rosenbaum AH. Anti-depressant treatment of the pain-prone disorder. Psychopharmacol Bull 1984; 20:531–535

[25] Turk DC, Salovey P. Chronic pain as a variant of depressive disease: a critical reappraisal. J Nerv Ment Dis 1984; 172:398–404

[26] Williams JMG. The psychological treatment of depression. A guide to the theory and practice of Cognitive Behaviour Therapy, 2nd edn. London: Routledge 1996: 77–109

[27] Arroll B, Khin N, Kerse N. Screening for depression in primary care with two verbally asked questions: cross sectional study. BMJ 2003; 327:1144–1146

[28] Beck, Steer, Brown. The Beck Depression Inventory 1996 (BDI-II), 1996

[29] Main CJ, Wood PL, et al. The distress and risk assessment method. Spine 1992; 17(1):42–52

[30] Zigmond AS, Snaith RP. The Hospital Anxiety and Depression Scale. Acta Psychiatrica Scan 1983; 67:361–370

[31] Beck AT, Ward CH, et al. An inventory for measuring depression. Arch Gen Psychiatry 1961; 4:561–571

[32] Pincus T, Williams A. Models and measurement of depression in chronic pain. J Psychosom Res 1999; Sep 47(3):211–219

[33] Spivey N. Enduring creation: art, pain and fortitude. Thames and Hudson, 2001

[34] Padfield D. Perceptions of pain. Verona: EBS, 2003

[35] Flor H, Turk DC. Chronic low back pain and rheumatoid arthritis: predicting pain and disability from cognitive models. Journal of Behavioural Medicine 1988; 11:251–265

[36] Nicholas MK. Self-efficacy and chronic pain. Paper presented at the annual conference of the British Psychological Society, St Andrews, 1989

[37] Rosensteil AK, Keefe FJ. The use of coping strategies in chronic low back pain patients; relationship to patient characteristics and current adjustment. Pain; 1983;17:33–44

[38] Flor HR, Turk DC, Rudy TE. Relationship of pain impact and significant other reinforcement of pain behaviours; the mediating role of gender, marital status and marital satisfaction. Pain, 1989; 38:45–50

[39] Krir J. The importance of psychosocial aspects in clinical assessment. British Journal of Chiropractic 2001; 4(2-3):50–53

[40] Harl, NJ, Georgieff K. Development of the Coping Strategies Questionnaire 24, a clinically utilitarian version of the Coping Strategies Questionnaire. Rehabilitation Psychology 2003; 48(4):296–300

[41] Williams DA, Thorn DE. An empirical assessment of pain beliefs. Pain 1989; 36(3):351–358

[42] Williams AC. Facial expression of pain: an evolutionary ACCOUNT. Behaviour Brain Science 2002; 25(4):439–455

[43] Waddell G. A new clinical model for the treatment of low back pain. Spine 1987; 12:632–644

[44] Fishbain DA, Cole B, Cutler RB, Lewis J, Rosomoff HL, Rosomoff RS. A structured evidence-based review on the meaning of nonorganic physical signs: Waddell signs. Pain Medicine 2003; 4(2):141–181

[45] Prkachin KM, Schultz I, Berkowitz J, Hughes E , Hunt D. Assessing pain behaviour of low-back pain patients in real time: concurrent validity and examiner sensitivity. Behaviour Research and Therapy 2002; 40(5):595–607

[46] Asghari A, Nicholas MK. Pain self-efficacy beliefs and pain behaviour. A prospective study. Pain 2001; 94(1):85–100

[47] Roland M, Morris R. A study of the natural history of back pain Part I: development of a reliable and sensitive measure of disability in low-back pain. Spine 1983; 8:141–144

[48] Flor H. Cortical reorganisation and chronic pain: implications for rehabilitation. J Rehabil Med 2003; May(41 Suppl):66–72

[49] Marhold C, Linton SJ, Melin L. Identification of obstacles for chronic pain patients to return to work: evaluation of a questionnaire. J Occup Rehabil 2002 Jun; 12(2):65–75

[50] Parloff M. Frank's common elements' in psychotherapy: non-specific factors and placebos. American Journal of Orthopsychiatry 1996; 56:521–530

[51] Beck AT. Cognitive therapy as the integrative therapy. Journal of Psychotherapy Integration 1991; 1(3):191–198

[52] Beck AT, Rush AJ, Shaw BF, Emery G. Cognitive therapy of depression. New York: Guildford Press, 1979

[53] Turk DC. Cognitive-behavioural approach to the treatment of chronic pain patients. Reg Anae Pain Med 2003; 28(6):573–579

[54] McCracken LM, Gross RT. Does anxiety affect coping with chronic pain? Clin J Pain 1993; Dec 9(4):253–259

[55] Borkovec TD, Robinson E, Pruzinsky T, DePree JA. Preliminary exploration of worry: some characteristics and processes. Behav Res Ther 1983; 21:9–16

[56] Eccleston C, Crombez G, Aldrich S, Stannard C. Worry and chronic pain patients: A description and analysis of individual differences. European J Pain 2001; 5:309–318

[57] Wells A. Cognitive therapy of anxiety disorders. Chichester: Wiley 1997

[58] Bortz WM. The disuse syndrome. West J Med 1984; Nov 141(5):691–694

[59] Crombez G, Vlaeyen JW, Heuts PH, Lysens R. Pain-related fear is more disabling than pain itself: evidence on the role of pain-related fear in chronic back pain disability. Pain 1999; 80(1-2):329–339

[60] Hale AS. ABC of mental health: anxiety. BMJ 1997; 314:1886

[61] Clark DM. A cognitive model of panic. Behav Res Ther 1986; 24:461–470

[62] Dehghani M, Sharpe L, Nicholas MK. Selective attention to pain-related information in chronic musculoskeletal pain patients. Pain 2003; 105(1-2):37–46

[63] McCracken LM, Eccleston C. Coping or acceptance: what to do about chronic pain? Pain 2003; Sep 105(1-2):197-204

[64] Derbyshire SW, Vogt BA, Jones AK. Pain and Stroop interference tasks activate separate processing modules in anterior cingulate cortex. Exp Brain Res 1998; 118(1):52–60

[65] van Tulder MW, Ostelo RWJG, Vlaeyen JWS, Linton SJ, Morley SJ, Assendelft WJJ. Behavioural treatment for chronic low back pain. Cochrane Database of Systematic Reviews 2003; 3

[66] Durand MJ, Loisel P. Therapeutic return to work: rehabilitation in the workplace. Work 2001; 17(1):57–63

[67] Merskey H, Bogduk N. International Association for the Study of Pain Classification of Chronic Pain: descriptions of chronic pain syndromes and definitions of pain terms. Pain 1986; 3:S1–S226

[68] Blazer DG, Kessler RC, McGonagle KA, Swartz MS. The prevalence and distribution of major depression in a national community sample: the national comorbidity survey. Am J Psychiatry 1994; 151:979–6

[69] Gilbert P. Depression: the evolution of powerlessness. Hove: Lawrence Erlbaum 1992

[70] Harris S, Morley S, Barton SB. Role loss and emotional adjustment in chronic pain. Pain 2003; 105(1-2):363–370

[71] Sullivan MJL, Reesor K, Mikail S, Fisher R. The treatment of depression in chronic low back pain: review and recommendations. Pain 1992; 50:5–13

[72] Ingram RE, Miranda J, Segal ZV. Cognitive vulnerability to depression. New York: Guildford Press, 1998

[73] Pincus T, Morley S. Cognitive-processing bias in chronic pain: a review and integration. Psychol Bull 2001; Sep 127(5):599–617

[74] Young JE. Cognitive therapy for personality disorders: a schema focused approach. Sarasota Professional Resource Press, 1990

[75] Young JE, Klosko Reinventing your life: how to break free from negative life patterns. Plume 1992

[76] Epston D, White M. Narrative means to therapeutic ends. London: Norton, 1990

[77] Radley A. Making sense of illness. London: Sage Publications, 1994

[78] Corbin J, Strauss AL. Accompaniments of chronic illness: changes in body self biography and biographical time. In: Roth JA, Conrad P, eds. Research in the Sociology of Health Care Vol 6, The Experience and Management of Chronic Illness. Greenwich, Conn.: JAL Press, 1987

[79] Schiaffino KM, Shawaryn MA, Blum D. Examining the impact of illness representations on psychological adjustment to chronic illness. Health Psych 1998; 17(3):262–268

[80] Lillrank A. Back pain and the resolution of diagnostic uncertainty in illness narratives. Soc Sci Med 2003 Sep; 57(6):1045–1054

[81] Safran JD, Segal ZV. Interpersonal processes in cognitive therapy. USA: Basic Books, 1990

[82] Imura S. Transference and countertransference in nursing. Emphasis Nursing 1991; 1:77–81

[83] Nesse RM , Lloyd AT. The evolution of psychodynamic mechanisms. In: Barkow JH, Cosmides L, Tooby J, eds. The adapted mind: evolutionary psychology and the generation of culture. Oxford: OUP; 1992: 601–624

[84] Obholzer A, Roberts VZ. The unconscious at work. Individual and organisational stress in the human services. London: Routledge:1997

[85] Winnicott DW. Hate in the countertransference, in Collected Papers: through paediatrics to psycho-analysis. London: Hogarth Press and the Institute of Psychoanalysis; 1958

[86] Lloyd Williams M, Payne S. A qualitative study of nurses' views on depression in palliative care patients. Pall Med; 2002

Many of the preceding chapters have dealt with the neuroscience and neurophilosophy of sensation and pain. These processes were all but absent in the chapter on psychosocial factors, which described the impact of pain on the individual as a person. It is the brain where these mental and emotional processes combine with the physiology. Sensory input influences the way the brain deals with pain, and so does psychology. The brain may be the place where the Cartesian division between body and mind is beginning to dissolve most clearly.

It is not the intention of the author to present the reader with a complete text on the brain and pain. Instead, models and observations that can be of use to the physical therapist are presented. An attempt is made to link the processes that form the physiological basis of nociception and pain with cognitive and emotional factors. These interactive processes are all viewed from an overarching model, in which the brain is seen as the central scrutinizer. The brain's function is to monitor and regulate. It is able to change sensation and it has an influence over most if not all bodily functions. Therefore, therapists ought to try to get the brain on board, either prior to or along with a physical intervention. No brain, no gain.

PAIN AND ATTENTION

By its very nature, pain demands attention. It is a signal indicating that something is wrong and that action may be required. However, human beings have the option of exerting their free will and deciding whether or not they pay attention to a pain. Long distance runners get used to feeling and analyzing pains. A new pain may require a change in running style or indicate the end of the race. On the other hand, the runner may decide that it is not worth acting on it and focus attention on other things. The redirection of attention soon makes the awareness of the pain disappear.

The example of the long distance runner demonstrates that attention can be manipulated in order to reduce the impact of pain. Redirection of attention is therefore a strategy that patients with persistent pain can use. An important requirement for the success of this approach is the presence of an alternative object of attention. This object needs to be important to the individual. In the case of the marathon runner, completion of the run or winning the competition has to be important. If he does not care about these things, there is a good chance that awareness of physical discomforts keeps building up, until the brain eventually decides to stop the activity.

Patients attending pain management programmes (PMPs) are asked to make a list of activities that they would like to take up or return to. These activities have to be meaningful to them as a person, so that they can be used as a new focus of attention. The PMP then sets about enabling patients to acquire the necessary physical and psychological tools to work towards these goals. Patients are encouraged to focus on functional measures such as walking distance or the ability to sit. It is hoped that when the patient leaves the PMP, the functional gains will translate into the ability to work, study or have a

---

Box 7.1 Patient example: the use of functional goals as distraction

Peter developed persistent low back pain, which eventually forced him to give up his work as maintenance engineer. X-rays and scans did not show any significant abnormality and treatments were no more than a brief glimmer of hope. Now Peter spent most of his days at home. Most of his friends had been colleagues and he gradually lost touch with them. The pain made it impossible to concentrate on anything else.

When Peter was first seen at the PMP, the clinicians at the programme had to force him to think of functional goals. 'I just want to get rid of the pain, that's all,' he would say. Through their encouragement and insistence, Peter eventually began to remember the interest in paintings that he used to have before his career took over his life. He bought some art books and found that he was able to ignore the pain while he was distracted.

Peter decided that he would like to rekindle his old interest further by going to college. Together with the therapists, he worked out what the physical demands would be. For example, he would have to be able to sit for long enough to finish a task in class. The therapists incorporated a graded programme that included tolerance to sitting, ways of introducing breaks and healthy ergonomics. Peter began to go out more, continued to develop his interest and rebuilt his social life, all of which helped to distract him from his pain.

leisure activity (see Box 7.1). This approach constitutes a redirection of attention, away from the pain.[3]

Attentional control of pain can also be conceptualized as redressing the balance between internal and external focus. Pain draws attention inwards. Some patients with persistent pain develop hypervigilance, an excessive awareness of internal body sensations. This internal focus may become so powerful that it interferes with the demands of the world around the patient, who withdraws, loses concentration and becomes irritable. Most treatment strategies that utilize attention attempt to redirect it to external elements.

Thanks to modern imaging techniques that enable brain activity to be mapped while a physical and/or psychological intervention is used (Box 7.2), it is now clear that distraction has a genuine effect on the brain. When distraction is used successfully to reduce pain, there is a decreased activation of brain structures involved in the response to pain.[4] In addition, pain controlling centres in the brain are activated when a person is distracted from a painful stimulus.[5] In other words, the psychological intervention has neural correlates.

An approach to pain control that seems diametrically opposed to distraction, is the use of deliberate attention. Some patients learn to control their pain by concentrating on it (Box 7.3). Flor et al asked amputees with phantom limb pain to make a mental effort to differentiate location and frequency of non-painful of electrical impulses delivered to the stump.[7] In other words, they were asked to deliberately focus on sensations arising from the painful area. This intervention reduced phantom limb pain, which is notoriously difficult to treat. Flor et al were also able to show that it also reverted changes in representation of the limb in the brain's cortex (see Cortical representation below). As with distraction, research investigating brain activation suggests that pain control through concentration is related with changes in brain activation.

It is interesting to note that changes in brain representation have also been found in patients with persistent low back pain.[8] It is therefore possible that attention to the symptomatic area can be used to reduce the impact of musculoskeletal pain.

Another use of deliberate attention is the so-called *mindfulness* approach, which involves relaxation and the unconditional acceptance of any sensation that arises.[9] Rather than teaching clients to turn away from the pain, it asks them to mentally scan the body in a deliberate and systematic way. The client is asked to be aware of sensations without attaching labels to them or taking action against them. This approach has been utilized effectively in the reduction of pain and intake of analgesics, with associated improvements in mood and activity.[10,11]

It is interesting to see that two seemingly contradictory interventions can have the same result. In summarizing the literature on attention, Hasenbring hypothesizes that both attention focusing and distraction move attention away from *the emotional reaction* to pain, rather than the pain itself.[12] As a result, both methods have the potential to reduce the impact of the pain.

Box 7.2 Pain imaging techniques

Modern pain imaging techniques have made it possible to visualize which parts of the brain are activated, both by pain and by therapeutic techniques.[6] These techniques are beginning to show how cognitive factors, such as the expectation of pain and distraction, can change the brain's reaction to pain.

The most recent development in the identification of brain structures involved in the perception and modulation of pain is brain imaging. Brain activity cannot be made visible directly, but some of the physiological changes associated with it can. For example, it is known that synaptic activity is associated with an increased metabolic rate of glucose. By using radioactive labelling of glucose, this metabolism can be shown with *Positron Emission Tomography* (PET) or *Single Photon Emission Computed Tomography* (SPECT). Other physiological changes related to the activation of brain regions are oxygen consumption and blood flow. These processes can be visualized using *functional Magnetic Resonance Imaging* (fMRI). These modern imaging techniques enable researchers to identify which brain structures are activated in response to certain types of pain, but also when physical and psychological interventions are used.

Box 7.3 Patient example: control of headaches using concentration

Bob has frequent headaches. They can be controlled with medication, but the side effects make it hard to concentrate and interfere with Bob's work. However, Bob has discovered a different technique. He sits in a quiet place and relaxes his body. When he feels relaxed, he begins to concentrate on the area of pain in his head. He tries to feel exactly where the pain is and what it feels like, in as much detail as possible. After a few minutes, the painful area begins to diminish. Eventually it is reduced to a small sphere of a few square millimetres in diameter. Once this has been achieved, a normal painkiller is sufficient to extinguish the pain completely.

Comparison of the two strategies however, suggests that distraction is the least effective method.[12] This may be because if the pain continues despite the distraction, it serves as a perpetual reminder that the coping strategy is not working, thereby inducing more distress. In addition, distraction may create a conflict between the central scrutinizer's tendency to pay attention to pain and the patient's efforts to ignore it. The patient's cognitive attempts at ignoring the pain may therefore increase the brain's efforts to amplify nociceptive input. In comparison, deliberate focusing enables the brain to analyse sensory information, after which it can reduce its sensory input back to a normal level. Attention to the painful area enables a patient to maximize normal sensation and not just pain. This can be compared to the way normal movement and sensory input are used in physiotherapy for stroke patients.[13]

Distraction may be a successful strategy in laboratory research trials,[4] but this success does not necessarily carry over into real life. Research subjects are protected by stringent ethical regulations and can withdraw from a research trial at any time. The pain is induced artificially and will not last. As a result, the emotional component of the pain, which Hasenbring feels is an important factor, is not present in most laboratory-based research. The central scrutinizer will allow attention to be directed at will, but only in the absence of stimuli that are potentially important to the individual.

The reason that distraction is utilized successfully in PMPs is likely to be explained by the context provided by those programmes. Patients are given detailed explanations of the origins of their pains. Seemingly unpredictable alterations of the pain are made more understandable. The patient learns that the pain does not represent a threat to the body's integrity. In other words, the central scrutinizer is assured that the pain does not require constant vigilance, so that it can begin to focus on the other things.

In conclusion, both attention and distraction can be used successfully in the management of pain. When selecting a strategy for a patient, it is important that an evaluation is made of the meaning of the pain for the patient. For example, if it represents fear, strategies involving distraction may be counterproductive because they go against the brain's tendency to be vigilant. Some of the tests discussed in Chapters 6 and 8 can help to predict how the central scrutinizer is interpreting and responding to the pain. Examples are the Fear Avoidance Beliefs Questionnaire and the Tampa Scale of Kinesophobia. Once the patient's fears have been addressed, distraction may be added as a strategy to control pain.

EXPECTATION OF PAIN

The description of the role of the nervous system quoted in the introduction to this chapter has an important shortcoming. It suggests that the regulatory role played by the brain is purely reactive. This suggestion has been challenged by Melzack's formulation of the neuromatrix model, which poses that the brain has its own blueprint of what the body should feel like (see Cortical representation below).[14] This brain map is *modified* but not *determined* by sensory input, as demonstrated by patients with phantom limb pain. Another indication that the brain does more than simply respond to sensations in an ad-hoc manner, lies in the observation that the pain experience is influenced or even generated by anticipation.[15]

Chapter 2 discussed the model of evolutionary development of the sensory nervous system and the value of detection of stimuli that may become noxious in the future. The ability to anticipate noxious stimuli can be seen as an evolutionary progression from the ability to merely respond to them. Getting away from an animal that has bitten you is useful, but avoiding the encounter is even better. The ability to do this relies on the brain's capacity to store and recall circumstances and the results of previous actions.

The perception of pain and its unpleasantness is associated with activity in certain areas of the brain. The interested reader may wish to refer to a review by Treede et al for a discussion of the brain regions that are activated by painful stimuli.[16] Recent research has shown that anticipation determines the strength of response in those areas. For example, if a painful stimulus is given to the subject in a predictable way, the brain's response is not very strong.[17] However, if the same stimulus is delivered in an unpredictable way this response is much stronger. In addition, the anticipation of unpredictable pain also increases the response to unpredictable stimuli that are not painful.[18] In other words, pain-related uncertainty enhances the effect that stimuli have on the central nervous system, so that even innocuous sensations can trigger a 'panic response' in the brain.

As discussed in previous chapters, there are several mechanisms that decrease the predictability of persistent pain. For example, peripheral neuropathies can cause paroxysms of pain. Neuropathic pain may also respond to a host of unrelated factors through the development of sensitivity to adrenaline and noradrenaline. Central sensitization can occur when nociceptive stimulation persists, changing the pain response even further and making the pain seem to have a mind of its own. In other words, pain related changes are associated with increasing levels of unpredictability. This unpredictability is likely to enhance the brain's response, not only to the pain but also to sensations that are not painful.

Explaining why a pain arises and why it behaves the way it does reduces uncertainty and should be part of any pain treatment; this author has been thanked by many patients, simply for taking time to explain the symptoms. For some, this clarity was all they needed to get the pain under control and return to activity. This is confirmed by emerging evidence, which suggests that a detailed explanation of pain physiology is capable of changing both physical performance and pain-related psychological changes in patients with persistent low back pain.[19,20]

Anticipation of pain does not only enhance the brain's response, it can also enhance the transmission of nociceptive impulses in the dorsal horn. Anticipation has been shown to activate cells in the dorsal horn before the painful stimulus is delivered.[21] This activation is mediated by nerves that descend from the brain stem to each spinal level,[22,23] which also play a role in the development of secondary hyperalgesia and neuropathic pain.[24] It has been suggested that this activation may even be sufficient to *create* pain in absence of painful stimulation.[15]

Although much is as yet unknown, the relevance of the information above can be summarized as follows. Neural pathways from the brain can facilitate the way nociceptive information is processed in the spinal cord. Activation of these pathways may enhance or create pain and can contribute to the development of persistent pain states. One factor that has to be shown to activate descending facilitation is the expectation of pain, so anticipation of pain may cause or maintain pain.

The fact that the brain may amplify sensations when it expects pain may not make immediate sense if pain is regarded as a negative phenomenon that needs to be combated. However, the interpretation of the brain as central scrutinizer explains that it is in the brain's interest to predict pain. It therefore enhances the input from the relevant channels, so that correct action can be taken as soon as possible. The unfortunate side effect of this strategy is that hypothetically pain may be generated in absence of nociception. Fortunately, clinicians can counter this self-generated pain by increasing predictability and by introducing a realistic expectation of pain relief.

ANTICIPATION OF PAIN RELIEF

Not only is the anticipation of pain associated with the facilitation of nociception, the anticipation of relief can often be enough to create relief.[25] The model of the brain as central scrutinizer offers a way of conceptualizing this interesting phenomenon. Pain informs a person that something is wrong and forces them to take action. Generally, the unpleasantness of pain and the consequences of tissue damage drive people to try to achieve a pain free state.[26] When steps are taken to remove pain and/or its cause, the scrutinizer no longer needs to pay attention to it. In order to avoid the pain distracting from more important tasks, the brain starts to suppress pain perception. This is similar to drinking in order to quench thirst. As soon as water has been taken in the thirst disappears, even though the water will take longer to be absorbed. The brain simply has no need for the sensation of thirst any more. Based on this principle, even physically ineffective treatments can achieve a result, although the efficacy tends to wear off on repetition.

The link between expectation and the relief of pain has been investigated extensively and is usually referred to as placebo analgesia. For a review of the literature, see Price's books on the psychology of pain and its relief.[27,28] The fact that patients visit clinicians with the expectation of an answer to their physical problems means that therapeutic encounters are inextricably linked with placebo effects. The increasing influence of science on medicine has led to the idea that treatments

Box 7.4 Difficulties in determining the influence of the placebo effect on symptoms

Scientific evaluation of the efficacy of a physical treatment relies on the manipulation of well-controlled treatment variables and separating those from psychological influences. However, other factors influence the observed results, which can then be falsely attributed to either the intervention or the influence of the patient's mind. Apart from the placebo effect, the following factors have to be taken into account when dealing with clinical (as opposed to experimental) pain.[31]

Natural history. Symptoms often wax and wane of their own accord. Figure 7.1A illustrates the natural fluctuation of symptoms. Even an ineffective treatment can be perceived to either worsen or improve symptoms, simply because of its timing.

A treatment that makes matters worse can be perceived as beneficial (Fig. 7.1B) and an effective treatment can seem to be detrimental (Fig. 7.1C). Because most patients seek help when their symptoms are reaching a peak, many interventions have a high chance of success (obviously this does not necessarily apply in situations where long waiting lists exist).

Regression to the mean. If symptom levels are set against the frequency that they occur, the results are likely to conform to a normal distribution (Fig. 7.2). This means that an average symptom level is most common, while extreme levels are relatively rare. The patient is likely to seek help when symptoms are extreme, even though they are likely to make room for more moderate ones.

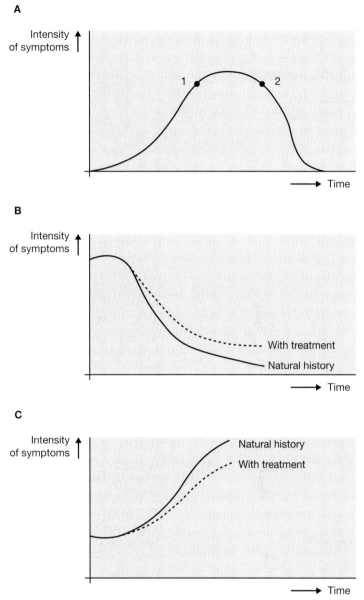

Fig. 7.1 The effects of natural history on the evaluation of a treatment. **A.** The symptoms produced by a condition fluctuate naturally. An ineffective intervention at point 1 has no benefits, because the symptoms continue to increase. The same intervention at point 2 is perceived to be beneficial. **B.** The natural improvement is slowed down by a treatment. Because the symptoms still improve, the treatment appears to be effective. **C.** A treatment is effective in slowing down the natural increase in symptoms, but cannot stop or reverse it. The continued increase falsely suggests that the treatment makes the symptoms worse.

continued

continued

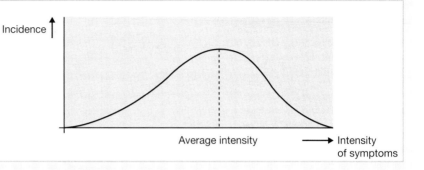

Fig. 7.2 Symptom levels are plotted against incidence over a long period, producing a bell shaped curve. Symptom levels are likely to return to a moderate level, because it is most common.

have a physiological component as well as a psychological element.[29] Bioscientists prefer to separate the physiological from the non-physiological effects of a treatment, because they regard only the physical effects as genuine.[30] As a result, to many the term placebo has become synonymous with quackery and deception.

Unfortunately for scientists, all cognitive and emotional processes associated with an intervention seem capable of influencing its efficacy, sometimes to a high degree.[31] Even the seemingly neutral information in a consent form can bias the results of a clinical trial. The Cartesian separation of body and mind may therefore be applied to highly artificial situations, for example when a drug is administered without the awareness of the patient. However, it has very little relevance for therapeutic encounters in real life, especially where hands-on treatments are concerned. Past experience, associations and personal interaction are inextricably linked with the outcome of a therapeutic encounter. In addition, natural fluctuation of symptoms may be falsely interpreted as a consequence of a treatment (Box 7.4).

It may not be ethical to subject a patient to an ineffective treatment in order to manipulate their psychology and achieve an effect based purely on their expectation. However, there is considerable scientific evidence that placebo analgesia involves the activation of pain controlling systems within the central nervous system. Not making use of these powerful systems in order to maximize the patient's chances of overcoming their pain could be regarded as equally unethical. The following section discusses the science of endogenous analgesia, which should help the reader to make an informed decision concerning this moral dilemma.

ENDOGENOUS OPIOIDS AND DESCENDING INHIBITION

Anticipation of pain relief has an analgesic effect, which is mediated by physiological systems. In other words, the mind is able to control pain because the physiology enables it to do so. For example, the knowledge that a pain relieving drug is being administered, makes the relief greater than when the drug is given without the knowledge of the patient.[35] This added analgesic effect can be blocked completely by the administration of naloxone, a substance that inhibits the action of opioids.[36] This applies even when the pain relieving drug is not an opioid and suggests that placebo analgesia involves opioids that are produced within the body.

There are several centres in the brain that produce opioids. In turn, the release of opioids activates nerves that descend to the spinal cord to inhibit the transmission of nociceptive signals (Fig. 7.3).[37,38] Examples of these centres are the peri-aqueductal grey (PAG), locus ceruleus and the nucleus raphe magnus (NRM). In laboratory settings, their role in pain relief has been confirmed by observing the effects of electrical stimulation of these centres or a direct injection of morphine (which is also an opioid).[27]

The reader will recall the discussion of inhibitory interneurones in the dorsal horn (see p. 62). The nerves descending from the brain involved in the inhibition of pain activate this type of interneurones. In response, the interneurones will release an opioid that will inhibit the transmission of nociceptive signals. The opioid has an effect on both the presynaptic and the postsynaptic membrane. On the presynaptic membrane, the release of excitatory neurotransmitters is inhibited. The postsynaptic membrane is hyperpolarized and therefore less likely to generate an action potential. In other words, the release of opioids in the dorsal horn makes it less likely that neurotransmitters are released, while the ones that are released are less likely to trigger a response in the secondary nerve.

The three functional processing states of the dorsal horn discussed in Chapter 4 are control, sensitized and suppressed. It may now be clear that these states are determined by the descending influence from the brain, which acts directly on the transmission of nociceptive

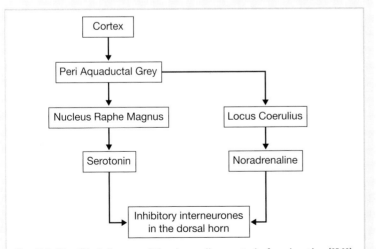

Fig. 7.3 Simplified diagram of the descending control of nociception.[37,38] Nerves from the para-aqueductal grey (PAG) connect with neurones in the nucleus raphe magnus (NRM) and locus coerulius (LC), which descend to the spinal cord. Here, they release serotonin and noradrenaline, which activate inhibitory interneurones.

Box 7.5 Rational therapies and the ethics of placebo treatment

It is a common misconception that a treatment that can be explained rationally does not rely on placebo effects. For example, the benefits from arthroscopic clearout and lavage of the knee joint can be explained by the perceived improvements in its biomechanical status. A joint is expected to move more easily and cause less pain after the removal of debris and the smoothing of the articular surfaces. However, a study comparing these treatments with placebo surgery found no differences between groups, either subjectively or functionally.[32] This suggests that although the influence of the mind is an inescapable reality of treatment, placebo controlled trials make clinicians re-examine and adjust the paradigms underlying assessment and treatment.

Is it ethical to apply placebo treatments? An article written in response to the aforementioned trial of knee arthroscopy questioned the ethics of subjecting patients to placebo surgery. It concluded that no treatment should be above scientific scrutiny.[33] Maureen Simmonds points out that patients turn to medical practitioners for treatments that are backed by science and not based on faith, but that it is unclear when the inevitable placebo becomes an instrument of deception.[29] Discussions on the development of quackery are offered by Jarvis[34] and www.quackwatch.com.

It is clear that expectation is a potent factor in the relief of pain. Its impact can be manipulated by the use of impressive equipment and the manner, appearance and reputation of the clinician. The paradoxical result is that the more a clinician tries to get away from the placebo effect by becoming an expert by using highly sophisticated techniques for examination and treatment, the greater is the contribution of the patient's mind to the efficacy of the treatment. By the same token, when the physical therapist stops taking the treatment itself seriously, it is likely that the treatment's efficacy will also reduce ...

Box 7.6 The model of the neuromatrix

The description of the role of the nervous system given at the beginning of this chapter suggests a reactive function: detection of events, evaluation and response. This makes it hard to understand phantom limb sensations, because the input that sets in motion the above process is absent. In an attempt to solve this paradox, Robin Melzack has put forward the concept of the neuromatrix.[14]

Melzack suggests that the brain contains processes that represent how a person's body feels to them. These processes form a neuromatrix, a blueprint of normal awareness. They are present whether sensory input is received or not. However, information from the body can modulate or trigger neuromatrix actions. In patients with amputations or other forms of nerve damage the moderating influence of some sensory input is reduced, leading to hyperactivity in parts of the central nervous system. This hyperactivity can be triggered by input from other areas, which are normally not associated.

This model has implications for the way physical therapies are practised. If pain is regarded as the consequence of input from the periphery, then it makes sense to focus the treatment on the body. However, the neuromatrix model suggests that pain can be interpreted as a result of a lack of normal input that moderates brain patterns, leading to the recruitment of different inputs that trigger abnormal patterns. It is therefore important that normal input is restored and that input that triggers abnormal responses is avoided. Note that this is not the same as avoiding pain altogether. Rather, it means that the sensory input created by the intervention does not raise the central scrutinizer's alarms, thus avoiding triggering abnormal central responses. An example from the author's practice is given in Box 7.8. Further suggestions concerning the application of neuromatrix principles have been put forward by Moseley.[48]

signals at a spinal level. This system can be activated by the expectation of pain relief. This is not a generalized effect on the whole spinal cord, but specific for the area of the body where relief is expected.[39] Another factor that activates descending inhibition under certain conditions is distraction.[5]

Another analgesic response that was discussed in previous chapters is associated with stress. For example, if a person is in a life-threatening situation, pain is often not felt until the immediate threat is over. This so-called stress induced analgesia is in part mediated by the descending inhibitory control system.[37] The PAG is under direct control of the hypothalamus, which integrates central pain control with the fight-or-flight response discussed in Chapter 5.[40]

CORTICAL REPRESENTATION

The cortex of the brain is the area where cognitive and emotional processes take place.[41] Different cortical regions deal with specific aspects of sensations, but there is also a high degree of integration.[42] Tactile, proprioceptive and emotional components of sensation are combined with information from other senses and memory.[43] One could say that the cortex is where sensory information is given meaning and where action is planned and instigated.

It is possible to construct a body map of a cortical area dealing with sensation. The earliest example of this type of map was developed by Wilder Penfield, who stimulated different areas of the cortex in awake subjects. He found that this stimulation produced sensations in the subjects' body, the location of which depended on the cortical region that was targeted.[42] With advancing technology, it has become possible to do the opposite by stimulating somatic regions and tracing which brain areas respond, as discussed above.

One of the most fascinating developments in recent years is the finding that cortical maps are highly adaptable (see Lundborg for an accessible review[44]). This is most obvious in amputees with phantom limb pain.[45] In these patients, the cortical region representing the amputated limb enlarges and becomes more easily excitable. Surrounding areas become able to trigger a response in this region. For example, upper limb amputees may find that tactile stimulation of the skin around the mouth can trigger sensations in the phantom arm, because cortical regions for the face and the hand are close to each other.[46]

A possible reason for this cortical reorganization is the formation of new synapses. In the example of the upper limb amputees, the neurones representing the face may form new synapses with neighbouring nerves that no longer receive peripheral input. However, this mechanism fails to explain how cortical representation can change very quickly in response to afferent activity.[47] It is becoming clear that widespread connections exist within the cortex, but that there is a high degree of *redundancy*, i.e. that a substantial proportion of these connections is usually not active. Cortical representation can therefore change quickly without requiring structural changes (Box 7.6).

The following experiment is suggested by the brain researcher Professor Ramachandran.[46] It does not always yield results, but when it does the change is quite remarkable. Persons A and B sit opposite each other (Fig. 7.4). A is wearing a blindfold and touches the nose of B, drawing circles around the tip of B's nose. C is standing behind A whilst drawing identical circles around A's nose. This provides A's brain with input that is similar to when A is touching his own nose. The reader is invited to carry out this experiment, preferably choosing a naïve subject for A's role, for 5–10 minutes. Before taking off A's blindfold, ask him how long he thinks his nose is and be prepared for an unusual answer ...

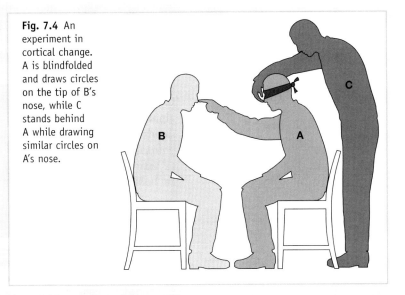

Fig. 7.4 An experiment in cortical change. A is blindfolded and draws circles on the tip of B's nose, while C stands behind A while drawing similar circles on A's nose.

The changes in cortical response that are found in patients with phantom limb pain can also take place as a result of peripheral nerve damage.[49] For example, carpal tunnel syndrome is associated with reorganization in several areas of the central nervous system and a heightened brain response, even to stimulation of the *ulnar* nerve.[50] Interestingly, cortical changes have also been found in patients without frank nerve damage, for instance those suffering with non-specific low back pain[8] or CRPS Type I.[51,52] This has been compared with the facilitation of synaptic links that forms the basis of learning and memory.[45] It is possible that this adaptive process in the brain maintains persistent pain by increasing responsiveness. This exaggerated response may be triggered by painful input from the affected area, but also by normal sensations from other body regions.

These findings beg the question how a physical therapist can meaningfully influence a patients pain. Herta Flor and her team devised a sensory discrimination regime, in which patients were asked to discriminate the frequency and location of electrical stimuli applied to the stump.[7] The effect was a significant reduction in both phantom limb pain and cortical reorganization. This suggests that deliberate attention to non-painful input may help to normalize cortical representation. Other methods designed to change cortical mapping are mental practice and the use of mirrors, which gives the visual impression of normal appearance and movement by mirroring the unaffected side (Fig. 7.5). Evidence supporting the use of these therapies is beginning to emerge.[53,54]

Taken together, the research findings discussed here suggest that pain syndromes are likely to involve changes of cortical representation. These changes may form a 'pain memory' that can be triggered by stimuli that are not necessarily painful in themselves. In other

- Does the patient avoid activities as a result of the pain?
- Does the patient persist in activities despite the pain?
- Does the patient adopt unusual postures in response to the pain?
- Has the patient developed altered movement patterns because of the pain?
- If the patient uses aids such as sticks, crutches, a wheelchair, belts or bandages, are they likely to be of benefit?
- If the patient is taking medication, are they exceeding the maximum doses?
- The use of functional measures advocated in Chapter 8 can be helpful when assessing the impact of pain on general activities. For example, the patient may be able to perform at a certain level in the clinical environment, but do less well at work as a result of perceived risks. The Fear Avoidance Beliefs Questionnaire and the Tampa Scale of Kinesophobia together with the findings from the physical examination may suggest that the brain's response to sensory input is inappropriate.
- If the behavioural response generated by the brain is the most appropriate way that the person can cope with their pain, then this suggests that the brain's analysis of the problem and its response are optimal. When this is the case, the clinician's priority is likely to be to address the cause of the pain.
- Inappropriate behaviour in response to pain may be the result of a lack of understanding of its origin. A well-known example is the patient with back pain, who lies supine most of the day because he thinks that the pain indicates a further crumbling of the vertebrae. The only way out of the situation in which lack of activity and muscular support maintain the pain, is the introduction of graded exercises and activities. This is likely to incur some pain, usually without damage. As long as the patient is convinced that crumbling of the spine causes the pain, the chance of cooperation with a rehabilitation programme is minimal. In fact, forcing the patient to go along with the suggestions of the therapist is likely to heighten the alertness of the central scrutinizer, leading to exaggerated reactions to even the slightest of stimuli.
- It is recommended that the therapist invite the patient to explain exactly what they think the pain indicates. It is important to keep an open mind and accept what the patient says. It must be remembered that the patient's understanding is influenced by past experience, emotions, family history and the responses of people around them. This understanding may not be rational, but that is not to say that the patient is stupid or malingering. Most people generate the best possible response based on their own cognitive and emotional makeup. It is the task of the clinician to uncover what underlies that response, and to modify it with compassion if required. Helpful questions can be 'What do you think is causing the pain?' or 'What is the best explanation you have been given for this pain?'
- Attention to pain and the emotional response generated by pain are governed by the amount of concern that the patient has regarding its

nature. This is one of the major differences between pain and mere nociception. It is therefore worth finding out how much concern the pain generates. For example, the clinician may ask 'What do you think would happen if you ignored the pain and did more?' or 'How do you think you will be in 10 years' time?' The pain scales published by the British Pain Society ask not only about the level of pain, but also about the emotional response to the pain. These scales can be downloaded as PDF files from http://www.painsociety.org/pain_scales.html

- As mentioned earlier, uncertainty heightens the alertness and responsiveness of the nociceptive system. As a result, bewilderment regarding the origin of the pain is likely to be detrimental to the patient's progress. In the author's experience, this is common in patients with low back pain of insidious onset, but also in patients with neurogenic pains that seem to behave in inexplicable ways. The scrutinizer may try out all sorts of responses without consistent benefit. It may also become increasingly unfocussed in an attempt to make some sense out of the pain, sensitizing increasing sections of the nervous system in the process and ultimately making matters worse.

- The reader is referred back to the assessment section of Chapter 4 for ways of determining whether the dorsal horn is in a sensitized state. In that chapter, state dependent processing was presented as a relatively autonomous phenomenon. However, this chapter has explained how the dorsal horn state is in fact determined by descending influences from the brain to a large extent. Therefore, when there is evidence of referred pain and other changes suggestive of central sensitization, it is likely that the central scrutinizer has reason to amplify or maximize its sensory input. Identifying these reasons and addressing them can be an important strategy in the management treatment of pain. This applies equally to situations where a causative lesion can be identified.

- Brain lesions are often associated with pain. Examples are central post-stroke pain and pain as a result of Parkinson's disease and multiple sclerosis.[56] The exact mechanisms underlying this type of pain are as yet unclear. It is important to query a history of neurological signs and symptoms, especially in older patients.

- Patients with a history of treatment failure may not expect to get better when the next clinician and clinical situation trigger the same responses as before. As discussed, the expectation of relief activates the endogenous opioid system. This activation is also linked to conditioning.[57] Therefore, being in the same or a similar environment as where treatment failure occurred, or being treated by the same person or with the same methods, is unlikely to trigger endogenous pain control.

- This does not mean that the patient has to be tricked into believing that the next clinician is a miracle worker who will fix the problem. What it does mean, is that the clinician who is confronted with a patient who has tried many things before can get the patient's own pain controlling system to cooperate by avoiding cues that may trigger old learned responses. If it is known where the patient was seen before, it may be worth seeing the patient in a different room, wearing different clothes and using a different approach. It may

Box 7.8 A neuromatrix approach to physical therapy

Paula was a 25-year-old teacher who presented with a 10-year history of widespread pain. This had started with an illness that required a month of bed rest. Paula developed neck ache, which gradually spread to the left arm and the entire back. All medical tests were negative and a range of treatments in the form of manual therapy, acupuncture, medication and injections had failed to bring relief.

Paula kept the pain at bay by keeping busy, but experienced increased pain if she did too much. She was in a lot of pain whenever she could not do much. Other aggravating factors were light touch, lack of sleep and stress. Paula did not understand why her body hurt so much and was terrified. She admitted that she tended to search for a diagnosis in periods that were relatively comfortable, while frantically searching for relief whenever the pain increased. The therapist observed that Paula kept changing position while sitting, leaning over to either side. Paula explained that she was getting away from the pain.

Neuromatrix analysis: the scrutinizer is on high alert, because there are persistent signals of threat that are not understood. Distraction suppresses these signals but also increases the risk of overuse, so once the distracting task is finished the brain response is even stronger. Leaning away from the painful side may temporarily bring relief, but ultimately creates ongoing abnormal input into the neuromatrix, thereby triggering abnormal responses.

Treatment: a detailed explanation of pain mechanisms, especially sensitization in the central nervous system, as well as principles of activity pacing and the importance of normal (albeit limited) postures and movements. The patient was asked to pace activities that were important in her daily life such as standing, sitting and preparing food. She was also asked to limit her periods of rest. Over the following weeks, her pain reduced. Gentle stretching exercises were introduced with close attention to the sensation they created, in order to

continued

help to explain to the patient that the idea is to start from scratch and explore any gaps in the previous treatments. Ask the patient to talk about previous treatments and assessments and try to get an impression of what they were comfortable with.

Similarly, it may be possible to make use of cues that the patient associates with relief. This does not mean that merely imitating a helpful situation is ethical or even sufficient, but it is a matter of adapting one's style to the patient. The big names in various types of therapy are reported to do this naturally.[58] The explicit use of these cues is the basis of Neuro Linguistic Programming (NLP).

- It is difficult to assess cortical representation in the clinical setting. However, it is possible get an impression by asking a patient to describe how the affected body region feels to them with their eyes closed. This is easier for the limbs and head than for the trunk. The patient is asked to focus on sensations of length, thickness, temperature and texture, as opposed to pain. They are also asked to compare with the unaffected side, if applicable. Another assessment tool that this author uses is the mirror therapy (Fig. 7.5). Some patients experience a reduction in pain when they are presented with the image of a normally functioning body part.

It must be stressed that the strategies suggested here are based on a model that views the brain as the central scrutinizer, in charge of monitoring and control. An understanding of this model enables the clinician to generate therapeutic strategies addressing sensory processing and behaviour, without having to become psychologists.

TREATMENT

Once the examination has been completed, the clinician should be able to answer the following questions:

- What are the likely sources of nociceptive input into the brain?
- What are the pain mechanisms involved?
- If it is not possible to explain all signs and symptoms, what is the most likely hypothesis?

Please note that this discussion is limited to the brain in the current discussion, so clinical considerations such as Red Flags are not mentioned here.

Next, the answers to these questions can be compared with the patient's insight into the cause and nature of the pain, ways they have tried to deal with their symptoms and the impact of the pain on their function. For a realistic assessment of function that does not rely purely on impressions formed in clinic, the use of objective functional outcome measures is strongly recommended (Ch. 8). The following questions should be answered:

- Is the patient's insight realistic and helpful?
- Are the patient's responses to their symptoms appropriate?
- Is the impact on the patient's function in line with their physical problems?

continued

The aim of this approach is to identify gaps between the central scrutinizer's analysis of and response to the pain on the one hand, and the reality as seen by the therapist. It is important that this gap is bridged, in order to align the efforts of clinician and patient. This can be achieved by giving a patient a realistic explanation of their signs and symptoms. In many patients with persistent pain, the mechanical model is often insufficient when trying to explain how and why symptoms behave the way they do and why treatments fail to bring lasting relief. It is therefore recommended that the explanation includes peripheral and central pain mechanisms. There is evidence of correlation between the patient's understanding and their physical function[19] and the importance of pain education alongside physical intervention.[20] However, if the therapist's knowledge is insufficient to generate adequate hypotheses, the involvement of an expert is essential.

The patient ought to be encouraged to ask questions about the explanatory model offered by the clinician. Appropriate explanations given to the patient in the past, either by professionals or lay people can be reinforced. However, overly simplistic and defective information from other sources has to be countered or moderated, so that the patient is not left with conflicting bits of knowledge. Some patients need to be offered some time to consider the new model that they are presented with and some like to check information for themselves. It may be helpful if the clinician can recommend some textbooks, articles or websites that chime with the message given to the patient (Appendix 7).

The intended effect of these discussions is to reduce the alarm state of the central scrutinizer. Clear understanding of the pain and the way it behaves helps to reduce anxieties concerning possible undetected pathologies and normalizes the brain's response. It also makes the pain more predictable; another factor in determining the way the brain reacts. This can only be successful if the patient feels that they are taken seriously and that the therapist has some compassion for them. Patients may describe behaviours that seem bizarre, but simply confronting them is unlikely to help. Instead, the therapist has to uncover how the current situation has developed and help the patient to share these insights.

Distraction can be a useful tool in the control of pain, but not until the above process has been completed. If the mind is not put at rest regarding the nature of the pain, distraction is likely to increase anxiety and raise the scrutinizer's vigilance. However, once these issues are addressed, distraction can be used in the form of mental exercises and the return to activities that are meaningful to the patient.

The neural processes underlying persistent pain conditions are similar to those underlying learning (see Box 4.4). Any sensory triggers similar to the ones that caused or maintained the pain have the potential to activate the neural pathways involved in the pain. Therefore, these triggers must be avoided at first and then gradually reintroduced. On the other hand, normal input should be maximized by using non-noxious sensory stimulation, normal movement, distraction and pleasant environments.

familiarize Paula with the sensory input created by normal movement. Great efforts were made to help her distinguish between acceptable sensations such as muscle stretch and sensations that could be a threat.

Progression: graded increases in activity and introduction of more functional postures and movement. Postural correction was started with the back against the wall. The wall provided a sense of safety and postural feedback, while the legs were kept slightly bent to strengthen their muscles. When Paula felt comfortable doing this and her confidence in her strength had increased sufficiently, standing away from the wall was practised. Eventually this was progressed to bending down and lifting.

Example of neuromatrix element of progression: once Paula began to get control of her lumbar posture, she started to experience an ache between her shoulder blades. The therapist examined her. He did not find any abnormalities, but only some muscular tenderness. He explained that the flattened lumbar lordosis forced the thoracic muscles to work a bit harder in order to reduce the compensatory kyphosis. He pointed out that this was therefore a sign of progress and that the thoracic ache could be used as a postural feedback tool, at least until the muscles strengthened.

Outcome: after a total of seven treatments spread over 10 weeks, the patient felt well enough to go travelling. Her therapist reinforced the self-management principles that Paula had learned and added advice for flights and bus journeys. Paula returned a few months later. She had experienced some pains, but had felt in control and not alarmed. She had been able to stay active and did not feel that further input was needed. She did however feel ready to reduce her drug intake and was referred to a Nurse Practitioner in pain management for advice.

CONCLUSION

The descending inhibitory system is activated when the brain no longer needs to pay attention to the pain. Confidence in the therapist, expectation of relief, reduction of fears and anxieties associated with the pain and acceptance are factors that play a role in this activation. On the other hand, as long as the central scrutinizer remains on alert, it maximizes and responds to any input that may possibly be of importance. The advice regarding the avoidance of cues that trigger unhelpful responses given in the assessment section, applies here as well. The patient who is given the impression that their current visit is a repetition of previous unhelpful experiences, either consciously or subliminally, is unlikely to activate their inhibitory systems.

There is a discrepancy between the views of the body based on modern science, which is devoid of meaning, and the brain's actions, which are based entirely on meaning. Pain manifests in the brain and is modified and acted upon by the brain, based on the meaning it attaches to it. Therefore, any treatment of pain has to take this evaluative process into account.

Finally, there is evidence that general exercise positively influences function and survival of the brain, so the restoration of physical function is important for a healthy central nervous system.[65]

Paradoxically, approaches that encourage body awareness can also be successful. This can be interpreted as a neuromatrix approach that opens the gates to normal input into the brain. Examples of these approaches are Mindfulness, Tai Chi and Chi Kung, Feldenkrais and Alexander.[9,59–62]

An important factor in any of these approaches and pain management approaches is the avoidance of threatening factors.[48] The patient should start off with an amount of activity that they are certain they can cope with. This activity has to be measurable in terms of duration, number of repetitions, distance, weight etc. For example, sitting may bring on a patient's pain after 15 minutes. Ten minutes is manageable, but begins to bring on some concern because the pain is expected to come on soon. The patient may say that 7minutes is fine. This baseline is recorded and the patient begins to sit for seven minutes regularly. This increases physical tolerance, but also reduces the element of threat by not exceeding limits that are safe according to the central scrutinizer. This approach is known in pain management programmes as *pacing*.[63,64] It is important that the exercises or activities that are chosen are meaningful to the patient.

Progression takes place by introducing a minute increment every day. The increase has to be small so that it does not trigger the brain's alarm reactions. For instance, the patient may introduce 10 extra seconds of sitting time every day. Other ways of introducing change is sitting on different chairs, or in different locations.

An example of neuromatrix physical therapy is given in Box 7.8.

References

[1] Amaral D. The anatomical organisation of the central nervous system. In: Kandel E, Schwartz J, Jessell T, eds. Principles of neural science. New York: McGraw-Hill, 2000: 317–336

[2] Gifford L. Pain, the tissues and the nervous system: a conceptual model. Physiotherapy 1998; 84(1):27–36

[3] Harding V, Williams ACdC. Extending physiotherapy skills using a psychological approach: cognitive-behavioural management of chronic pain. Physiotherapy 1995; 81(11):681–688

[4] Petrovic P, Ingvar M. Imaging cognitive modulation of pain processing. Pain 2002; 95(1,2):1–6

[5] Valet M, Sprenger T, Boecker H, et al. Distraction modulates connectivity of the cingulo-frontal cortex and the midbrain during pain – an fMRI analysis. Pain 2004; 109(3):399–408

[6] Casey K, Bushnell M. Pain Imaging. Seattle: IASP Press, 2000

[7] Flor H, Denke C, Schaefer M, Grusser S. Effect of sensory discrimination training on cortical reorganisation and phantom limb pain. The Lancet 2001; 357:1763–1764

[8] Flor H, Braun C, Elbert T, Birbaumer N. Extensive reoganization of primary somatosensory cortex in chronic back pain patients. Neurosci Lett 1997; 224:5–8

[9] Kabat-Zinn J. Full catastrophe living. How to cope with stress, pain and illness using mindfulness meditation. London: Piatkus, 1990

[10] Kabat-Zinn J. An outpatient program in behavioural medicine for chronic pain patients based on the practice of mindfulness meditation: theoretical considerations and preliminary results. General Hospital Psychiatry 1982; 4:33–47

[11] Kabat-Zinn J, Lipworth L, Burney R. The clinical use of mindfulness meditation for the self-regulation of chronic pain. Journal of Behavioral Medicine 1985; 8(2):163–190

[12] Hasenbring M. Attentional control of pain and the process of chronification. Progress in Brain Research 2000; 129:525–534

[13] Carr J, Shepherd R. The adaptive system: plasticity and recovery. In: Carr J, Shepherd R, eds. Neurological rehabilitation-optimizing motor performance. Oxford: Butterworth Heinemann, 1998: 3–22

[14] Melzack R. From the gate to the neuromatrix. Pain 1999; (Supplement 6):S121–S126

[15] Fields H, Basbaum A. Central nervous system mechanisms of pain modulation. In: Wall P, ed. Textbook of pain. Edinburgh: Churchill Livingstone, 1999: 309–329

[16] Treede R, Kenshalo D, Jones A. The cortical representation of pain. Pain 1999; 79(2,3):105–112

[17] Hsieh J, Stone-Elander S, Ingvar M. Anticipatory coping of pain expressed in the human anterior cingulate cortex: a positron emission tomography study. Neurosci Lett 1999; 262:61–64

[18] Sawamoto N, Honda M, Okada T, Hanakawa T, Kanda M, Fukuyama H et al. Expectation of pain enhances responses to nonpainful somatosensory stimulation in the anterior cingulate cortex and parietal operculum/posterior insula: an event-related functional magnetic resonance imaging study. J Neurosci 2000; 20(19):7438–7445

[19] Moseley G. Evidence for a direct relationship between cognitive and physical change during an education intervention in people with chronic low back pain. European Journal of Pain 2004; 8(1):39–46

[20] Moseley G. Combined physiotherapy and education is efficacious for chronic low back pain. Australian Journal of Physiotherapy 2002; 48:297–302

[21] Duncan G, Bushnell M, Bates R, Dubner R. Task-related responses of monkey medullary dorsal horn neurons. J Neurophysiol 1987; 57(1):289–310

[22] Ren K, Dubner R. Descending modulation in persistent pain: an update. Pain 2002; 100(1,2):1–6

[23] Porreca F, Ossipov M, Gebhart G. Chronic pain and medullary descending facilitation. Trends Neurosci 2002; 25(6):319–325

[24] Ossipov M, Lai J, Malan T, Vanderah T, Porreca F. Tonic descending facilitation as a mechanism of neuropathic pain. In: Hansson P, Fields H, Hill R, Marchetti P, eds. Neuropathic Pain: Pathophysiology and Treatment. Seattle: IASP Press, 2002: 107–124

[25] Price D, Milling L, Kirsch I, Duff A, Montgomery G, Nicholls S. An analysis of factors that contribute to the magnitude of placebo analgesia in an experimental paradigm. Pain 1999; 83(2):147–156

[26] Moseley G. A pain neuromatrix approach to patients with chronic pain. Manual Therapy 2003; 8(3):130–140

[27] Price D. Psychological mechanisms of pain and analgesia. Seattle: IASP Press, 1999

[28] Price D, Bushnell M. Psychological methods of pain control: basic science and clinical perspectives. Seattle: IASP Press, 2004

[29] Simmonds M. Pain and the placebo in physiotherapy – a benevolent lie? Physiotherapy 2000; 86(12):631–637

[30] Hart C. The mysterious placebo effect. Modern Drug Discovery 1999; 2(4):30–40

[31] Turner J, Deyo R, Loeser J, von Korff M, Fordyce W. The importance of placebo effects in pain treatment and research. JAMA 1994; 271:1609–1614

[32] Moseley J, O'Malley K, Petersen N, et al. A controlled trial of arthroscopic surgery for osteoarthritis of the knee. N Engl J Med 2002; 347(2):81–88

[33] Horng S, Miller F. Is placebo surgery unethical? N Engl J Med 2002; 347(2):137–139

[34] Jarvis, WT. Why health professionals become quacks. Online available: www.quackwatch.com 11-12-1998

[35] Amanzio M, Pollo A, Maggi G, Benedetti G. Response variability to analgesics: a role for non-specific activation of endogenous opioids. Pain 2001; 90(3):205–215

[36] Laurence D, Bennett P. Clinical pharmacology, 7th edn. Edinburgh: Churchill Livingstone, 1992

[37] Basbaum A, Jessell T. The perception of pain. In: Kandel E, Schwartz J, Jessell T, eds. Principles of neural science. New York: McGraw-Hill, 2000: 472–491

[38] Willis W, Westlund K. Neuroanatomy of the pain system and of the pathways that modulate pain. J Clin Neurophysiology 1997; 14(1):2–31

[39] Benedetti F, Arduino C, Amanzio M. Somatotopic activation of opioid systems by target-directed expectations of analgesia. J Neurosci 1999; 19(9):3639–3648

[40] Millan M. Descending control of pain. Prog Neurobiol 2002; 66:355–474

[41] Kandel E. The brain and behaviour. In: Kandel E, Schwartz J, Jessell T, eds. Principles of neural science. New York: McGraw-Hill, 2000: 5–18

[42] Amaral D. The functional organisation of perception and movement. In: Kandel E, Schwartz J, Jessell T, eds. Principles of neural science. New York: McGraw-Hill, 2000: 337–348

[43] Saper C, Iversen S, Frackowiak R. Integration of sensory and motor function: the association areas of the cerebral cortex and the cognitive capabilities of the brain. In: Kandel E, Schwartz J, Jessell T, eds. Principles of neural science. New York: McGraw-Hill, 2000: 349–380

[44] Lundborg G. Brain plasticity and hand surgery: an overview. J Hand Surg 2000; 25B(3):242–252

[45] Flor H. The functional organization of the brain in chronic pain. Prog Brain Res 2000; 129:313–322

[46] Ramachandran V. Phantoms in the brain. London: Fourth Estate, 1998

[47] Calford M. Dynamic representational plasticity in sensory cortex. Neuroscience 2002; 111(4):709–738

[48] Moseley G. A pain neuromatrix approach to patients with chronic pain. Man Ther 2003; 8(3):130–140

[49] Chen R, Cohen L, Hallett M. Nervous system reorganization following injury. Neuroscience 2002; 111(4):761–773

[50] Tinazzi M, Zanette G, Volpato D, et al. Neurophysiological evidence of neuroplasticity at multiple levels of the somatosensory system in patients with carpal tunnel syndrome. Brain 1998; 121:1785–1794

[51] Juottonen K, Gockel M, Silen T, Hurri H, Hari R, Forss N. Altered central sensorimotor processing in patients with complex regional pain syndrome. Pain 2002; 98(3):315–323

[52] Rommel O, Gehling M, Dertwinkel R, Witscher K, Zenz M, Malin J et al. Hemisensory impairment in patients with complex regional pain syndrome. Pain 1999; 80(1,2):95–101

[53] McCabe C, Haigh R, Ring E, Halligan P, Wall P, Blake D. A controlled pilot study of the utility of mirror visual feedback in the treatment of complex regional pain syndrome (type 1). Rheumatology 2003; 42:97–101

[54] Moseley G. Graded motor imagery is effective for long-standing complex regional pain syndrome: a randomized controlled trial. Pain 2004; 108(1,2):192–198

[55] Waddell G, Main C. Illness behaviour. In: Waddell G, ed. The back pain revolution. Edinburgh: Churchill Livingstone, 1998: 155–172

[56] Boivie J. Central pain and the role of quantitative sensory testing (QST) in research and diagnosis. Eur J Pain 2003; 7(4):339–344

[57] Amanzio M, Benedetti F. Neuropharmacological dissection of placebo analgesia: expectation-activated opioid systems versus conditioning-activated specific subsystems. J Neurosci 1999; 19(1):484–494

[58] Bandler R, Grinder J. The structure of magic. A book about language and therapy. Palo Alto, California: Science and Behaviour Books, 1975

[59] Reid H. The book of soft martial arts. Finding personal harmony with Chi Kung, Hsing I, Pa Kua and T'ai Chi. London: Gaia, 1988

[60] Chuen L. The way of energy. Mastering the Chinese art of internal strength with Chi Kung exercise. London: Gaia, 1991

[61] Feldenkrais S. Bewusstheit durch Bewegung. Der aufrechte Gang. Frankfurt am Main: Suhrkamp, 1978

[62] Barlow W. The Alexander principle. London: Victor Gollancz, 1991

[63] Harding V, Williams ACdC. Extending physiotherapy skills using a psychological approach: cognitive-behavioural management of chronic pain. Physiotherapy 1995; 81(11):681–688

[64] Harding V, Watson P. Increasing acitivity and improving function in chronic pain management. Physiotherapy 2000; 86(12):619–630

[65] Cotman C, Berchtold N. Exercise: a behavioral intervention to enhance brain health and plasticity. Trends in Neuroscience 2002; 25(6):295–301

Assessment of function

The definition of insanity is continuing to do the same thing over and over again, expecting a different result.

ALBERT EINSTEIN

INTRODUCTION

The assessment of function using standardized tests facilitates objectivity and evaluation of the treatment.[1] Evaluation of a patient's functional ability demonstrates the impact and the relevance of a person's pain on their lives. This is illustrated in the example given in Box 8.1.

This chapter reviews methods of functional assessment that are currently available and discusses the benefits of each to enable the clinician to select the most appropriate for specific applications. The relationship between function and pain is considered, including some factors that mediate between pain and function, such as fear and self-efficacy.

The benefits and limitations of the various approaches to assessing function are examined. Specific measures that have particular relevance for musculoskeletal clinicians are discussed. The chapter concludes with some considerations and recommendations for the selection and use of functional assessment measures.

FUNCTION AND IMPAIRMENT

Impairment has been described as a pathological or anatomical loss, or abnormality of a structure, or the physiological loss of function of a structure.[2] In the current text, the term *loss of function* relates to the individual, not to tissues (please refer to Box 8.2 for definitions of terms relating to function).

Traditional musculoskeletal objective assessment identifies impairments. It is often assumed that there is a linear causal relationship between impairment and loss of function. As a result, the patient may be treated with the expectation that the resolution of the impairment or tissue dysfunction will restore normal overall function and resolve disability.[3] However, there is a growing body of evidence of a very poor correlation between function and impairment.[4,5] For example, Simmonds et al illustrate that lumbar flexion, which is a measure of

Mrs A presents with low back pain. She reports the pain intensity as 8 out of 10 on sitting. The importance of this to her is that it is too painful to sit down long enough to watch television, drive a car or sit at her workstation. It is not just the pain, but also the loss of function that determines how much her back pain makes her suffer. The therapist who wishes to assess the impact of the pain has to have a way of measuring function. The evaluation of functional gains provides a measure of the relevance of therapeutic gains for the patient's life.

impairment, is extremely poorly related with measures that emulate lumbar functional activities.[5] They conclude that 'the issue is how patients move rather than how far they move'.

In a study looking at a new measure to determine recovery in patients with low back pain, Williams notes that clinicians' predictions of likelihood of return to work is only moderately correlated with the patients' own predictions.[6] This is due to the fact that the clinicians' ratings are a composite measure of impairment derived from their physical assessment, whereas the patients' concern is the effect on their function. Unfortunately, interventions that focus on impairments are not guaranteed to affect function.

FUNCTION, PAIN AND BELIEFS

As discussed in Chapters 6 and 7, the impact of pain on a person's function is in part determined by their perception of what that pain represents. For example, a person who believes that they have a lumbar disc that has literally slipped out of its natural position may also believe that each pain is a sign of further slippage. In that person's mind, every pain represents another step, away from possible recovery and closer to the operating table. Their predicament is quite different from that of someone who has decided that their back pain is part of the natural aging process. The pain is felt, may require some minor adjustments in lifestyle, but is essentially not a big problem.

Emotions and beliefs are therefore important in the experience of pain and its impact, see Box 8.3. The ones that are most relevant to function, including fear, self-efficacy and coping strategies are discussed below.

FEAR OF PAIN AND FUNCTION

The term kinesiophobia has been used to describe 'a genuine but hitherto unrecognized variant of phobic disorder...a fear of physical movement resulting from a feeling of vulnerability to painful injury or reinjury'.[7] Others have used the term fear avoidance.[3,8] The fear or anticipation of pain is in itself sufficient to inhibit activity.

The behaviour observed in some chronic pain patients may be a response to fear, rather than to pain directly. This is the cognitive behavioural model of fear of movement/(re) injury illustrated in Figure 6.2. For instance, Crombez and Vlaeyen have found significant correlation between fear of movement or of reinjury and physical performance as measured by torque generated in three repetitions of maximal trunk flexion/extension.[9]

Gains in pain relief and reductions of impairment may not be integrated into a patient's life, if fear of pain is not addressed. Furthermore, it may stop the patient from participating in exercise programmes and other interventions if some pain is involved. When a patient withdraws from a treatment programme, the clinician ought to determine whether fears were discussed and addressed beforehand.

Self-efficacy and function

Bandura makes a case for the importance of self-efficacy as a way of explaining behaviours in patients.[10] He asserts that the concept explains why individuals of equivalent abilities perform at different levels. Self-efficacy is the belief an individual has in his or her abilities. This can also be described as self-confidence. Self-efficacy affects the effort that people put into an activity.

The therapist who identifies poor self-efficacy underlying a loss of function can assist the patient in changing that belief by providing evidence to the contrary. It is common for patients with persistent pain to focus on pain levels and not to notice functional gains. For example, a patient may state that their back pain is no better, but not realize that they have doubled their walking distance or sitting time. Functional outcome measures enable a therapist to take the focus of the treatment away from the pain and redirect it towards attainment of function.

Self-efficacy is important, because it determines how much a patient will be able to do despite the pain. This is particularly relevant if the pain cannot be taken away, for instance in patients with severe rheumatoid arthritis. In addition, activity can provide distraction from the pain. A pain sufferer who is able to go out or work has distractions, while someone who feels unable to do anything can only concentrate on their symptoms.

THE IMPORTANCE OF FUNCTIONAL ASSESSMENT

An individual's functional status is related to and yet distinct from their impairment. Therefore, the therapist cannot make assumptions about function based upon their evaluation of impairment alone. It is essential to make an assessment of the functional status of the patient an integral part of the assessment process.

Function is related to pain, yet the relationship is complex being mediated by beliefs and emotions. Functional assessment may therefore involve the identification of these beliefs and feelings. Methods that do this are included in the sections that follow.

Functional assessment introduces a higher level of objectivity into the assessment of patients. Pain assessment is often based on self-report from the patient, instead of objective assessment of the impact of the pain. The use of relevant functional outcome measures provides an objective way of evaluating the effectiveness of treatment, in a way that is relevant to a patient. Reliable and valid methods of assessing function are considered below. It is beyond the scope of this text to include all the measures available. The primary focus is on measures that are currently used in the study of patients with pain. Much attention is given to measures that are valid for the assessment of low back pain, because this is the area in which most work has been done to date. Other measures are specific to other anatomical regions such as shoulder or knee and some are more generic. The Chartered Society

Box 8.2 Definitions of terms used in this text*

Ability: the potential to do/ perform an action.

Activity: the execution of a task or action by an individual.

Activity limitation: difficulty the individual has in executing tasks.

Disability: any restriction or lack (resulting from an impairment) of ability to perform an activity in the manner or within the range considered normal for a human being. Loss of the potential to do.

Dysfunction: physiological loss of function.

Function: to do, to perform. The special action or physiologic property of an organ or other part of the body.

Functional limitation: restriction in activity that can be related to disability, impairment and/or emotions and beliefs.

Functional status: summarizes the function of the individual including the things that individual does and does not do.

Impairment: problems in body function and structure such as significant deviation or loss. Any loss or abnormality of anatomical, physiological or psychological structure or function.

Incapacity: lacking capacity to do.

Loss of function: loss of activity; not doing.

* Where possible these definitions are taken from the WHO ICIDH and ICF. Some other terms are included because their use is common amongst physical therapists even though they do not form part of the WHO classifications.

- **Patient population:** low back pain
  (acute and chronic).
- **Locale:** primary and secondary care.
- **Scoring:** 24 unweighted statements
  covering activities related to mobility,
  self-care and sleeping scored 0/1;
  higher scores represent greater loss of
  function.
- **Time frame:** 24h.

Availability

- No copyright.
- May be reproduced (Appendix 2,
  p. 203).
- Translated into 11 different
  languages.

Advantages

- Large number of studies looking at
  psychometric characteristics giving
  good results.
- Lots of comparative data for
  researchers.
- Minimum detectable change scores
  available.

Disadvantages

- Was developed for researchers
  investigating groups therefore may
  not allow enough specificity of
  response for the individual.
- Not validated for conditions other
  than low back pain.

Face and content validity

The range of the RMDQ is limited. It omits some aspects of physical function such as lifting, carrying, pushing and pulling. It primarily covers physical function although there are a couple of psychosocial items. This may be seen as both a strength and a weakness.[17] The strength is that the measure is unambiguous. It makes RMDQ useful for investigating the relationships between psychological and social factors and self reported physical functioning.[16,18–22]

Construct validity

RMDQ has moderately strong correlations with other measures of physical function including Oswestry, Quebec Back Pain Disability Scale, the physical subscales of SF36 and (not surprisingly given its derivation) SIP.[17] RMDQ is also correlated significantly with pain related fear as measured by Fear Avoidance Beliefs Questionnaire (FABQ) and Tampa Scale of Kinesiophobia (TSK).[9] There are differing views as to whether or not there is a correlation between RMDQ and pain intensity (measured by VAS). Crombez et al[9] report no correlation, but Beurskens[19] and Simmonds[5] have found a moderate relationship.

Simmonds[5] and Deyo[22] both report that RMDQ is moderately correlated to physical performance. This means that there are instances when self reported function differs from observed performance. In the clinical setting, it is important to consider the reasons why this is the case. For example, Mr I, who walks 50 metres unaided in the perceived safety of the clinic, may be unable to overcome his fear of tripping in the street outside and hence fall back on using his crutches. Careful investigation of a perceived discrepancy will lead to more appropriate management strategies that address his fears.

Bar a report of trivial correlation between RMDQ and lumbar flexion,[5] there is very little data on the correlation between physical impairment and RMDQ and this is again an area that merits further investigation.

Internal consistency

The internal consistency of RMDQ is very high. Cronbach's alpha has been estimated between 0.84 and 0.91.[17]

Reproducibility

The RMDQ is a measure designed to pick up change in the acute stage when change is actually expected to occur (for the vast majority of patients). This makes the test–re-test reproducibility problematic. If the interval between tests is too short there is a danger that the respondent remembers their previous answers. If too long then change is likely as low back pain is a changeable condition even over the course of a day. For example, bending over to put socks on is impossible on first rising but possible an hour later. For this reason it is important to state the interval of time for which test–re-test has been performed. Roland and Morris reported test–re-test scores of 0.91 for acute back pain patients tested at an interval of one day.[13] However, RMDQ has been used extensively with the chronic back pain population. Peat cites test–re-test scores of >8.3 for up to 3 weeks and Jensen et al[24] report 0.72 for chronic back pain patients tested at an interval of 39 days.[23]

Responsiveness

The ability of a measure to detect change when it has occurred is it's most important attribute.[25] RMDQ is a responsive measure.[19] In their original study Roland and Morris reported median scores for patients with acute low back pain in primary care of 11 on presentation, eight 1 week later and four 1 month later. If this is what one expects to see in an acute low back pain population then larger changes must be seen in order to infer an intervention effect for patients treated in this early period.

There has also been a study to determine the smallest change that is clinically significant (the minimum detectable change or MDC) by Stratford et al.[26] They note that this will vary according to the initial level of disability. They have computed conditional standard errors of measurement to estimate minimum levels of detectable change for every possible combination of pre- and post score. They conclude that the MDC at the 95% confidence level is 4–5 points. This means that the scale is not responsive to positive change for scores below 4 points (floor effect) or negative change for scores above 20 points (ceiling effect).

The Oswestry Disability Index

Context

The Oswestry Disability Index (ODI) is another self-report measure that is related to a specific location of pain, the low back. It contains statements are primarily about function and therefore is a measure of the individual's beliefs about what they can and cannot do. The measure is summarized in Box 8.7 and reproduced in Appendix 3.

Background and development

The ODI was developed from data collected from interviewing patients with chronic low back pain attending a specialist clinic. The patients were asked about what effect their condition was having on their daily activity. Version 1 was published in 1981[27] and a form revised by the Medical Research Council research group in 1986. This is the recommended version[23] although there is a further version published by the North American Spine Society (NASS).

Box 8.7 Summary of Oswestry Disability Index

- **Patient population:** low back pain (acute and chronic).
- **Locale:** primary and secondary care.
- **Scoring:**
  - respondent marks one of six statements in each of 10 sections relating to activities of daily living.
  - score is doubled to give %.
  - higher scores represent greater loss of function.
- **Time frame:** not specified.

Availability
- No copyright.
- May be reproduced (Appendix 3, p. 204).
- Translated into at least nine different languages.

Advantages
- Large number of studies looking at psychometric characteristics giving good results.
- Lots of comparative data for researchers.

Disadvantages
- Was developed for researchers investigating groups therefore may not allow enough specificity of response for the individual.
- Not validated for conditions other than low back pain.
- 6-point Likert scale makes completing and scoring more time consuming than RMDQ.
- Some evidence that less responsive than RMDQ for those with moderate functional loss.[17]

Box 8.12 Resumption of Activities of Daily Living Scale

- **Patient population:** low back pain (acute and chronic).
- **Locale:** primary and secondary care.
- **Scoring:** respondent estimates the extent to which they have resumed usual activities for at least 9 of 12 items on a 0–100% scale. Total score divided by number of items to give % resumption.
- **Time frame:** not specified.
- **Availability:** measure in original paper.

Advantages

- Original work suggests good psychometric characteristics including minimum detectable change score.
- Patients estimate a percentage of recovery of their normal function so the measure is always relevant to them.

Disadvantages

- Recent measure so no independent research to date.

This circumvents the need for the researchers to set a standard of what is normal making the measure applicable to respondents with a wide range of abilities. It is summarized in Box 8.12.

Background and development

The RADL is a recent measure (1998) developed by Canadian researchers, Williams and Meyers, to distinguish between recovery which is spontaneous and that which is attributable to a treatment intervention by using individual's perceptions of recovery.[6]

At the time, there was a need to evaluate the community clinic programmes that had been introduced by the Workers Compensation Board in Ontario in 1989. These programmes were early interventions (<70 days since onset) for workers with a soft tissue low back injury aimed at facilitating early return to work. Yet critics questioned whether intervention was effective at reducing time absent from work for attendees compared to non-attendees given the expected rate of spontaneous recovery. Williams and Meyers wanted to develop a tool that would allow them to compare low back pain patients' recovery with the expected prognosis of LBP across a range of functional indicators besides return to work. Williams and Meyers cite Nachemson's estimate that for every episode of LBP, 50% of LBP will have recovered by 2 weeks; 70% by 1 month and 90% within 3 months. Williams and Meyer developed the RADL in conjunction with the FACS, which is considered below under Other tests.

Face and content validity

Content validity can also be described as the discriminant ability of the scale, that is, the extent to which it discriminates between individuals who differ in the attributes you are attempting to measure. The authors found differences in the RADL scores of individuals who were working and those who were not. They also found that the scores of subjects rated by their clinician as able to return to work at completion of the programme were higher than those of subjects rated unable to return to work.

Construct validity

This term describes the ability of the assessment tool to measure the thing it purports to. This can also be described as convergent validity. It is assessed by looking at the relationship between the measure being studied and others in the field. The authors found moderate correlation with RMDQ and their other scale, FACS, which is a measure of self-efficacy. They also noted a moderate correlation between RADL scores and clinician's ratings of physical conditioning. (This was given as a composite percentage score for endurance, range of movement, muscle strength, locomotion and overall ability to perform functional activities.)

sible on first rising but possible an hour later. For this reason it is important to state the interval of time for which test–re-test has been performed. Roland and Morris reported test–re-test scores of 0.91 for acute back pain patients tested at an interval of one day.[13] However, RMDQ has been used extensively with the chronic back pain population. Peat cites test–re-test scores of >8.3 for up to 3 weeks and Jensen et al[24] report 0.72 for chronic back pain patients tested at an interval of 39 days.[23]

Responsiveness

The ability of a measure to detect change when it has occurred is it's most important attribute.[25] RMDQ is a responsive measure.[19] In their original study Roland and Morris reported median scores for patients with acute low back pain in primary care of 11 on presentation, eight 1 week later and four 1 month later. If this is what one expects to see in an acute low back pain population then larger changes must be seen in order to infer an intervention effect for patients treated in this early period.

There has also been a study to determine the smallest change that is clinically significant (the minimum detectable change or MDC) by Stratford et al.[26] They note that this will vary according to the initial level of disability. They have computed conditional standard errors of measurement to estimate minimum levels of detectable change for every possible combination of pre- and post score. They conclude that the MDC at the 95% confidence level is 4–5 points. This means that the scale is not responsive to positive change for scores below 4 points (floor effect) or negative change for scores above 20 points (ceiling effect).

The Oswestry Disability Index

Context

The Oswestry Disability Index (ODI) is another self-report measure that is related to a specific location of pain, the low back. It contains statements are primarily about function and therefore is a measure of the individual's beliefs about what they can and cannot do. The measure is summarized in Box 8.7 and reproduced in Appendix 3.

Background and development

The ODI was developed from data collected from interviewing patients with chronic low back pain attending a specialist clinic. The patients were asked about what effect their condition was having on their daily activity. Version 1 was published in 1981[27] and a form revised by the Medical Research Council research group in 1986. This is the recommended version[23] although there is a further version published by the North American Spine Society (NASS).

Box 8.7 Summary of Oswestry Disability Index

- **Patient population:** low back pain (acute and chronic).
- **Locale:** primary and secondary care.
- **Scoring:**
  - respondent marks one of six statements in each of 10 sections relating to activities of daily living.
  - score is doubled to give %.
  - higher scores represent greater loss of function.
- **Time frame:** not specified.

Availability

- No copyright.
- May be reproduced (Appendix 3, p. 204).
- Translated into at least nine different languages.

Advantages

- Large number of studies looking at psychometric characteristics giving good results.
- Lots of comparative data for researchers.

Disadvantages

- Was developed for researchers investigating groups therefore may not allow enough specificity of response for the individual.
- Not validated for conditions other than low back pain.
- 6-point Likert scale makes completing and scoring more time consuming than RMDQ.
- Some evidence that less responsive than RMDQ for those with moderate functional loss.[17]

Face and content validity

ODI has good validity. The original study showed that the scores for 25 patients who might reasonably be expected to improve with time did fall.[27] Beurskens also showed expected improvements occurring.[19]

The scale differs from RMDQ because rather than giving dichotomous, or yes/no responses, the patient is asked to choose which one of six possible statements is most true of them.

Construct validity

ODI is well correlated to RMDQ and SF36 and moderately correlated with VAS and the McGill pain questionnaire.[17]

Internal consistency

The internal consistency of version 2 is acceptable. Chronbach's alpha has been estimated between 0.76 and 0.87 in various studies.[17]

Reliability (reproducibility)

The ODI is subject to the same difficulties as RMDQ in terms of decreasing reliability over time, but has also been used extensively in the chronic pain population.

Responsiveness

Buerkens et al compared the responsiveness of the ODI with RMDQ.[19] Their conclusion was that ODI was less responsive to change as measured by the patient's own judgement although still very useful. Stratford notes that this will vary according to the initial level of disability and states that the ODI is especially useful where the respondent's initial score is high.[28]

Back Pain Functional Scale

Context

The Back Pain Functional Scale was recently developed by Stratford.[28] It was published in 2000 as an alternative to the RMDQ. Like the RMDQ, this is an example of a self-report measure that is related to a specific location of pain: the low back. It too asks specifically about function and therefore is a measure of the individual's beliefs about what they can and cannot do. It is summarized in Box 8.8 and reproduced in Appendix 4.

Box 8.8 Summary of the Back Pain Functional Scale

- **Patient population:** low back pain (acute and chronic).
- **Locale:** primary and secondary care.
- **Scoring:** respondent scores degree of difficulty performing in 12 areas of function using a 6-point Likert scale where 0 = unable to perform and 5 = no difficulty.
- **Time frame:** not specified.

Availability

- On application to the author: PW Stratford, School of Rehabilitation Science, McMaster University, 1400 Main Street West, Hamilton, Ontario, Canada LS81C7. (Appendix 4, p. 206.)

Advantages

- Good psychometric characteristics including values for minimum detectable change scores.
- More specific to the individual than RMDQ.
- Better able to detect change in those with little or substantial functional loss (i.e. a smaller ceiling and floor effect) than RMDQ.

Disadvantages

- Recent measure so no independent research to date.

Background and development

The authors intention was to formulate a tool specifically to assist the clinical decision making process, unlike the RMDQ or ODI which were designed with research using group studies. The scale uses self-report of performance in 12 areas of function, which may be affected by back pain.

Face and content validity

The researchers have looked at the ability of the scale to discriminate between different work status, smoking status and location of symptoms and found that it could do so.

Construct validity

There is a strong association between BPFS and RMDQ scores.

Internal consistency

Chronbach's alpha is 0.93 at the 95% confidence interval.

Reliability (reproducibility)

Test–re-test reliability using a sample of 28 patients with low back pain tested at first visit to physician, within 48 hours then at 1, 2 and 3 week followups yielded a score of 0.88. This compares favourably to 0.81 for RMDQ.

Responsiveness

The researchers administered both RMDQ and this scale to 153 patients attending clinics for physical therapy in Canada and the USA and found that the measure was somewhat better at detecting change in patients with pain of less than 2 weeks duration than RMDQ. They have concluded that it is a competitive functional status measure.

The Tampa Scale of Kinesiophobia

Context

The Tampa Scale of Kinesiophobia (TSK) is a self-report measure concerned with the respondent's beliefs about the meaning of the pain and specifically their fear of damage and re-injury if they move. It does not measure loss of function but gives a measure of kinesiophobia that might be the cause of a loss of function. Although developed for assessing pain specific fear in low back pain patients, the measure has been widely used in other patient populations such as fibromyalgia. It is summarized in Box 8.9.

Box 8.9 Summary of Tampa Scale of Kinesiophobia

- **Patient population:** Chronic and acute low back pain, fibromyalgia and possibly other chronic pain
- **Locale:** Primary and secondary care
- **Scoring:** Original scale has 17 items scored on a 4-point Likert scale from strongly disagree (1) to strongly agree (4). The total score is calculated after inversion of scores from statements 4,8,12,16 and higher scores represent greater fear of movement and/or re-injury. Patients considered at risk if score over 40 Short version has 13 items scored on the same 4-point Likert scale. No inversion of scores. Higher scores represent greater fear of movement and/or re-injury. Subscales of fear-avoidance (items 1,2,7,8,10,11,12,13) and harm (items 3,4,5,6,9).
- **Time frame:** Not specified, patients simply asked to score how 'you feel'.

Availability

- Scale reproduced in appendix of Vlaeyen et al 1995 j Vvlyen, Institute for rehabilitation research, Zandbergsweg 111, 6432 cc Hoensbroek, The Netherlands. (Appendix 5, p. 207.)

Advantages

- Moderate to good psychometric characteristics
- Identifies beliefs and emotions underlying a loss of function and therefore may help to plan appropriate intervention.

Disadvantages

- No available minimum detectable change scores
- Does not identify nature or extent of functional loss and so needs to be used in conjunction with a measure that does.

Background and development

Kori, Miller and Todd, the medical director, senior psychologist and clinical director of the pain management programme at Tampa General Hospital in Florida, coined the term kinesiophobia in 1990.[7] They use the term to describe 'a genuine but hitherto unrecognized variant of phobic disorder...a fear of physical movement resulting from a feeling of vulnerability to painful injury or reinjury' ([7] p. 37). The authors argue that a substantial subset of chronic pain patients are the victims of an insidious psychobehavioural process where initial adaptive avoidance of movement persists beyond healing time becoming maladaptive. The patients' fear or anticipation of pain is in itself sufficient to inhibit activity. The behaviour observed in chronic pain patients is a response to fear rather than to pain directly.

The Tampa scale is the measure these researchers developed to detect kinesiophobia. The scale consists of 17 items that are rated by the respondent on a 4 point Likert scale. Crombez et al[7] recommend that patients scoring more than 40 out of a possible 67 merit further investigation to determine what specific things they are afraid of.

The respondent is asked to either strongly disagree (1); somewhat disagree (2); somewhat agree (3) or strongly agree (4). In the original scale most of the statements express a kinesiophobic point of view, for example, 'I wouldn't have this much pain if there weren't something potentially dangerous going on in my body' and 'I'm afraid that I might injure myself if I were to exercise'. Recent factor analysis by Goubert et al[29] suggest that there are two subscales of fear-avoidance and harm that give the best fit of data from 2 samples. These researchers recommend that a shortened version of the scale be used, which omits the four adaptive coping statements (numbers 4,8,12,16) included in the original scale and it is the short form version which is appended to this chapter.

Face and content validity

Content validity describes the extent to which a scale does actually assess the intended attributes. Vlaeyen et al[30] showed good content validity.

Construct validity

In a study of patients with chronic back pain, Crombez et al found significant correlation of TSK with the Fear-Avoidance Beliefs Questionnaire (FABQ).[9] The study also showed that self-reported disability, measured by RMDQ, and negative affect were significantly correlated with TSK. Importantly, TSK was not correlated with pain intensity as measured by VAS confirming the original authors' contention that it is fear of provoking pain, rather than the current level of pain, that has most impact on function.

Internal consistency

The internal consistency of TSK of the original 17 item scale is high. Cronbach's alpha that determines how well a set of items measure a single construct has been measured as 0.76 in one study of 35 chronic back pain patients.[30] Swinkels-Meewisse et al found it to be 0.70 and 0.76 in 2 tests of a group of 176 acute back pain patients.[31] The authors noted that the internal consistency increases further if the adaptive coping statements are deleted and this is confirmed Goubert et al[29] who found Cronbach's alpha to be 0.8 in pooled data for 188 low back pain patients and 0.82 for 89 patients with fibromyalgia.

Reliability (reproducibility)

The relevant criterion for a self-report evaluative measure is the intra test (test–re-test) reliability that is the extent to which a procedure yields the same result on repeated trials under the same conditions.

Swinkels-Meewisse et al[31] found a substantial test–re-test reliability of 0.78 in their sample of acute back pain patients testing up to a maximum of 24 hours later.

Responsiveness

There are no studies of responsiveness for this measure.

The Fear Avoidance Beliefs Questionnaire

Context

The Fear Avoidance Beliefs Questionnaire (FABQ), like the TSK, assesses the fear of pain, movement and reinjury as they relate to physical activity and work. It is a measure about beliefs and emotion that impact on function. It is summarized in Box 8.10 and reproduced in Appendix 6.

Background and development

Lenthem used the term fear avoidance in 1983, in his explanation of the persistence of low back pain.[32] Waddell developed the idea arguing that 'fear of pain and what we do about it may be more disabling than the pain itself.[3] He went on to develop a scale with colleagues that was published in 1993.[8]

Principal components analysis yielded two subscales, work and physical activity. These are correlated but distinct.

Face and content validity

Swinkels-Meewisse et al found high concurrent validity between FABQ and TSK.[31]

Box 8.10 Fear Avoidance Beliefs Questionnaire

- **Patient population:** chronic low back pain and possibly other chronic pain.
- **Locale:** primary and secondary care.
- **Scoring:** patient scores16 items reflecting fear and avoidance related to physical activity and work. Median score is 15.
- **Time frame:** not specified, patients simply asked to score how 'you feel'.
- **Availability:** Measure in original paper (Appendix 6, p. 208).[8]

Advantages

- Moderate to good psychometric characteristics.
- Distinguishes between factors of work and physical activity.
- Identifies beliefs and emotions underlying a loss of function and therefore may help to plan appropriate intervention.

Disadvantages

- No available minimum detectable change scores.
- Does not identify nature or extent of functional loss and so needs to be used in conjunction with a measure that does.

- **Patient population:** low back pain (acute and chronic).
- **Locale:** primary and secondary care.
- **Scoring:** respondent estimates the extent to which they have resumed usual activities for at least 9 of 12 items on a 0–100% scale. Total score divided by number of items to give % resumption.
- **Time frame:** not specified.
- **Availability:** measure in original paper.

Advantages

- Original work suggests good psychometric characteristics including minimum detectable change score.
- Patients estimate a percentage of recovery of their normal function so the measure is always relevant to them.

Disadvantages

- Recent measure so no independent research to date.

This circumvents the need for the researchers to set a standard of what is normal making the measure applicable to respondents with a wide range of abilities. It is summarized in Box 8.12.

Background and development

The RADL is a recent measure (1998) developed by Canadian researchers, Williams and Meyers, to distinguish between recovery which is spontaneous and that which is attributable to a treatment intervention by using individual's perceptions of recovery.[6]

At the time, there was a need to evaluate the community clinic programmes that had been introduced by the Workers Compensation Board in Ontario in 1989. These programmes were early interventions (<70 days since onset) for workers with a soft tissue low back injury aimed at facilitating early return to work. Yet critics questioned whether intervention was effective at reducing time absent from work for attendees compared to non-attendees given the expected rate of spontaneous recovery. Williams and Meyers wanted to develop a tool that would allow them to compare low back pain patients' recovery with the expected prognosis of LBP across a range of functional indicators besides return to work. Williams and Meyers cite Nachemson's estimate that for every episode of LBP, 50% of LBP will have recovered by 2 weeks; 70% by 1 month and 90% within 3 months. Williams and Meyer developed the RADL in conjunction with the FACS, which is considered below under Other tests.

Face and content validity

Content validity can also be described as the discriminant ability of the scale, that is, the extent to which it discriminates between individuals who differ in the attributes you are attempting to measure. The authors found differences in the RADL scores of individuals who were working and those who were not. They also found that the scores of subjects rated by their clinician as able to return to work at completion of the programme were higher than those of subjects rated unable to return to work.

Construct validity

This term describes the ability of the assessment tool to measure the thing it purports to. This can also be described as convergent validity. It is assessed by looking at the relationship between the measure being studied and others in the field. The authors found moderate correlation with RMDQ and their other scale, FACS, which is a measure of self-efficacy. They also noted a moderate correlation between RADL scores and clinician's ratings of physical conditioning. (This was given as a composite percentage score for endurance, range of movement, muscle strength, locomotion and overall ability to perform functional activities.)

Internal consistency

Cronbach's alpha was 0.89 indicating high internal consistency.

Reliability (reproducibility)

The RADL was tested with 20 individuals at a mean interval of 1.8 days (range 1–5 days). All individuals confirmed that their condition was the same for both tests. The intra class correlation coefficient was high at 0.83.

Responsiveness

Williams and Meyer calculated that a change of 16 points on the 100-point RADL indicates a clinically important change.

Canadian Occupational Performance Measure

Context

The Canadian Occupational Performance Measure (COPM) uses self-report of performance in areas of concern to the patient as the outcome.[34–36] This client-centred approach generates an individualized measure of function. It is summarized in Box 8.13.

Background and development

The COPM was developed in the late 1980s in consultation with occupational therapists across Canada practising in all areas of their discipline. The therapist and client generate a problem list together during an assessment. This allows the consideration of environmental and role factors unlike most other measures that prescribe the functions to be considered. The researchers identify other advantages of the measure: it allows measurement of different objectives for intervention such as restoration of function or prevention of change; it facilitates engagement of the client in the therapeutic process from the outset. It must be noted, however, that the measure is relatively new and there is little data on validity and reliability.

Face and content validity

The content validity of a scale that uses the participant's own evaluation of problems is necessarily tautological. The important factor is whether the process allows identification of the most significant problems. In their study of 61 disabled individuals, McColl et al report that 75% find the COPM useful in identifying and rating their problems.[37] It is of note that a scant majority (53%) spontaneously report

---

Box 8.13 Canadian Occupational Performance Measure

- **Patient population:** anywhere client has sufficient skills to engage in the process (may exclude clients with learning difficulties or lack of motivation).
- **Locale:** primary and secondary care.
- **Scoring:** client and therapist identify tasks within the performance areas of self-care, productivity and leisure where there are problems. The problems are ranked on a 1–10 scale for importance, ability to perform and satisfaction with performance to give weighted scores.
- **Time frame:** not specified.

Availability

- Guidelines available from CAOT publications, Carleton Tech and Training Centre, Ste 3400, 1125 Colonel by drive, Ottawa, Ontario, Canada K1S 5RI.

Advantages

- Measure is tailored to the individual allowing a genuine patient centred approach.

Disadvantages

- Lack of data on psychometric characteristics.
- Might not be appropriate for comparing outcomes between individuals.

a problem previously identified during the problem identification session. The authors are not clear whether this is because the COPM is a superior or inferior tool for identifying problems to other techniques.

Construct validity

Ripat et al[36] made a comparison of the COPM with the Health assessment questionnaire with 13 participants diagnosed with rheumatoid arthritis and reported good correlation coefficients for similar activities on the scales.

Reliability (reproducibility) and Responsiveness

There is no published data on reliability; however, the measure was recently used in the context of a UK multidisciplinary pain management programme to identify problems of specific concern to a sample of 101 patients. Sixty different problems were identified, of which 45 were mentioned by nine or less of the respondents.[38] This implies a high degree of problem specificity, strengthening the case for individualized assessment.

Decreased walking tolerance was the most frequently reported problem being mentioned by 56%. The researchers found that one-third of participants reported improvements of greater or equal than 2 points on the scale but as there is no research yet into minimum detectable change scores it is not possible to say whether this is a significant finding.

SPECIFIC PERFORMANCE TESTS

Various researchers have identified a need for standardized tests of physical performance that relate to function in the chronic pain population.[5,11] A number of performance tests have been used with other groups of patients, for example in cardiac rehabilitation and respiratory disease, but their suitability for assessing function in patients whose primary complaint was pain has not been evaluated.

The lack of research into the relationship between observed performance and self-report has been discussed above. A performance test is a sample of an activity that is only an approximation to life as it really is for the individual. In an ideal world one would simply observe individuals in their own environment. As this is impossible for most clinicians an alternative is to 'sample behaviour under controlled conditions'.[11]

It is extremely important to control the conditions of the test because it is very likely that the artificiality of the environment will have an effect on the result. What is less certain is whether the individual being tested will tend to over or under perform but it is likely that they will exhibit a similar response to the environment on each occasion of being tested. By replicating the conditions of the test each time, one is controlling this factor as far as possible. This might necessitate performing the test at the same time of day on each occasion and certainly means using the same words to instruct the person on what to do. On the other hand the tests are straightforward to score with the agreement between different scorers or inter-rater reliability commonly reported as very high or perfect.[11]

The sections that follow describe some of the most commonly used performance tests, which have been selected because they have good psychometric characteristics. Each test is described individually because this facilitates use of an appropriate test in the purely clinical setting. The general advantages and disadvantages of performance tests compared with self-report measures are summarized in Box 8.14.

Walking tests

Background and development

Walking tests are a longstanding part of physical therapy assessment and tests have been devised for use with patients with a wide variety of conditions apart from pain.[5] Harding et al describe a 10-min walk test where the person walks between two points a known distance apart and the total distance is calculated.[11] They also test a 5-min version of this test. Another walking test that has recently been assessed for use with chronic pain patients is the Shuttle Walk Test.[39,40]

Methods

Harding's test is an endurance walk where the patient walks between two measured points, turning at each end. The instruction to the patient is to cover as much ground as possible in the time permitted. (They also add the caveat 'bearing in mind the demands of the journey home following assessment' p. 370.)

The Shuttle Walk Test is an incremental walking test that emulates the laboratory exercise test. It was developed in the field of cardiopulmonary function testing. The patient turns around cones placed 10 metres apart so that the course describes an oval shape. The test can be paced so that the patient keeps time with a series of audio signals reaching each cone at the next signal. The interval between these signals decreases so that the patient has to walk faster to reach the cone. It is a compound test of walking distance and walking speed. The test is completed when the patient can no longer continue to walk and is scored as a distance completed and time taken. The researchers also collected data on SaO_2, peak heart rate and perceived effort.

Face and content validity

This psychometric characteristic is tautological because all tests of physical performance inherently measure themselves. It is important to guard against assumptions on how the measured physical performance will impact on function, however. Compensatory strategies or aids may help to maintain function in the face of poor performance, for example Mrs J who has a 5-min walk distance of 50 metres is able to maintain the function of exercising her dog by throwing a ball for him to chase whilst she rests sitting on a bench.

Construct validity describes the ability of the assessment tool to measure the thing it purports to. It is usual to compare the tool against other established measures. With any physical performance test, however, the most important aspect is how relevant the test is to the patient's function. In the case of a walking test this is how far the walking in the test is related to the kind of walking the patient does normally. Consider Mrs K who habitually walks for an hour every day. She is easily able to walk for 10 min and therefore a ceiling affect limits the usefulness of a 5- or 10-min test.

Reliability

Good reproducibility has been established for the 10-min walk test[11] (Pearson correlation coefficient = 0.944 for 431 patients tested at an interval of 4–6 weeks. The 10- and the 5-min versions of the walk test are very highly correlated and so the shorter test can be recommended.

Simmonds et al use the 5-min version of the test in their comparative study of 45 subjects with low back pain and 48 pain free subjects[5]. They also ask the patients for a rating of perceived effort at the end of the test using the modified Borg scale. The researchers report good intra- and inter-rater reliability when testing 2 weeks apart. These results confound the view of some authors who have argued that there is a significant learning effect and that the test only becomes valid after two or more attempts.[41]

Finally, the shuttle walk test shows good test–re-test reliability at an interval of 1 week.[40] The researchers also report significant and strong correlations for the distance completed and peak heart rate. There are significant and moderate correlation of peak SaO_2 and peak Borg rating of perceived exertion.

Responsiveness

The clinical utility of a test is determined by the extent to which it captures clinically meaningful change in patient's performance. There is little outcome data reported on this for physical performance measures generally. Harding et al showed that there was a significant change in the distances walked by patients pre- and post treatment, which comprised participation in a 4-week full time pain management programme.[11]

Stand up tests

Background and development

Simmonds et al use a test of repeated sit-to-stand, arguing that this is a common task performed more slowly by those with low back pain and therefore a relevant indicator of functional status in this group.[5]

They advocate timing five repetitions of the sit-to-stand manoeuvre. Harding et al also advocate a repeated sit-to-stand task, in this case the number of repetitions performed in 1 or 2 min is counted.[11] The repetitions have the disadvantage of making the tests less representative of real life but both sets of researchers include sit-to-stand on the grounds that it is nonetheless an important functional activity.

Methods

Simmonds et al's version of the test requires the subject to rise to standing and return to sitting as quickly as possible five times.[5] The time is noted. Harding et al's version of the test differs in that the subject continues the activity at the pace they determined for 2 min.[11] They also tested a 1-min version.

Face and content validity

The sit-to-stand tests described capture data on the speed of movement. Another significant feature is the quality of the movement. This aspect is not captured by the test unless it is specifically noted or a video recording made. This maybe useful if the clinician decides that quality of movement is an important feature. There are no existing recommendations for quantifying such data although it might be possible to use a screening method developed for assessing pain behaviours.[42]

Construct validity

This is a major issue for a repeated sit-to-stand test as the task is not a close approximation of daily function and the clinician is left to infer the likely functional gains for an individual whose score improves. These gains might include greater ease of movement in standing up and other tasks that involve hip and knee flexion such as dressing or picking objects off the floor. The gains might also reflect on tasks that require improved quadriceps power such as stair climbing. It is important to check with the patient rather than make assumptions about the relevance of this test to their function.

Reliability

Simmonds et al report moderate reproducibility for their five repetitions test and argue that this might be a general feature of a high velocity, dynamic movement.[5] Harding et al report good reliability of both 2- and 1-min versions of the test (Pearson correlation coefficient = 0.938).[11]

Responsiveness

Harding et al have found substantial and highly significant improvement in pre- and post treatment test scores.[11] Other aspects of the

Table 8.2 Other physical performance tests that have been used for patients with pain

Test	Reference	Scoring	Reliability	Responsiveness
Balance	Harding et al 1995	Single leg time to first touch summed	Poor test–re-test	Poor
Distance walk	Simmonds et al 1995	Timed 50 feet walk at preferred speed	Good	Poor
Grip	Harding et al 1995	Mean of 3 scores on dynameter	Good	Poor
Lumbar flexion	Simmonds et al 1998	3 warm up movements followed by measured flexion with inclinometers over T12 and S1	Fair (but natural) diurnal variation makes timing of re-test important)	Fair
Peak flow	Harding et al 1995	Best of 3 scores on Wright mini-peak flow meter	Good	Fair (for pain management programme; good for respiratory function training)
Repeated trunk flexion	Simmonds et al 1998	10 reps timed	Poor	No data
Sit ups	Harding et al 1995	Max reps scored	Good	No data
Sorenson fatigue test (back extensor fatigue time)	Simmonds et al 1998	Time to fatigue to hold upper body horizontal in line with lower	Good	No data
Timed up and go	Simmonds et al 1998	Time to stand from a chair, walk forward 3 m and return to sit	Fair	No data

performance tests. They actually use a single repetition of a number of movements, which means that the therapist must infer the effects of impaired function from impairment.

Face and content validity

The tests involve the performance of eight movements with the participant rating their performance as good or poor for each movement according to a preset criterion. As measurements of impairment (in this case a loss of range of movement) the tests are inherently valid, yet the question remains to what extent the tests correlate either to real restrictions of function or to pain.

Construct validity

Hellsig analyses results from 834 respondents and find small but statistically significant differences in the test scores of respondents with no problems, moderate problems and severe problems.[4] There are small but significant differences in responses to fear of activity (as measured by 4 questions with a 6-point Likert scale), catastrophic thoughts and test scores.

Reliability

In a pilot study of 20 symptom free individuals, Hellsig has found 98% concordance between an observer's ratings and the individuals' ratings.[4]

Responsiveness

Hellsig has not reported any data on responsiveness. Linton, studying the benefits of a cognitive behavioural therapy intervention (CBT), has found a small deterioration in scores for the CBT group at 1-year follow up, indicating that impairments do not respond positively to CBT.[46]

References

[1] Petty NJ, Moore AP. Neuromusculoskeletal examination and assessment. A handbook for therapists, 2nd edn. Edinburgh: Churchill Livingstone; 2001

[2] World Health Organisation. WHO international classification of impairments, disabilities and handicaps ICDH. Geneva: World Health Organisation; 1980

[3] Waddell G. A new clinical model for the treatment of low back pain. Spine 1987; 12:632–644

[4] Hellsig A-L, Linton SJ, Bryngelsson IL. Eight simple, self-administered tests to add to symptom registration: a preliminary report. Spine 1997; 22:2977–2982

[5] Simmonds MJ, Olson SL, Jones S, et al. Psychometric characteristics and clinical usefulness of physical performance test in patients with low back pain. Spine 1998; 23:2412–2421

CONCLUSION

The relevance of pain, loss of movement or weakness to a patient is the effect it has on their function. It is therefore essential for physical therapists to make an assessment of function. This is particularly important for patients with chronic conditions, because gains in function offer ways of reducing the suffering associated with their pain.

Choosing an appropriate measure is vital but is by no means an easy task. The factors to consider are summarized in Box 8.14.

Self-report of function using a standardized questionnaire is used allows the individual to tell us about her own environment if it asks questions that are appropriate to them.

The responses given reflect the person's beliefs about their function. These beliefs may differ from observed performance. This makes it important to consider the collection of data on *both* self-report of function and observed performance of tasks. The careful investigation of any discrepancy between self report and observed performance can be achieved by direct questioning or by using measures which inform about the thoughts and feelings underlying a person's self reported functional status. This will lead to more appropriate management strategies.

The use of established measures is strongly recommended. This is important for patient care, but also for the evaluation of treatment efficacy by audit and research. In the case of low back pain the two recommended contenders are RMDQ and ODI and Peat[23] argues that anyone contemplating using any other measure should be able to demonstrate why neither of these two is adequate. Nevertheless, there is growing interest in measures that use the patients' own perception of their functional problems as outcome measures in order to improve relevance to the individual. The COPM and RADL are examples of such measures.

Functional assessment is an essential part of the assessment and management of patients and it is hoped that this chapter will help the physical therapist to ask relevant questions and make informed choices when selecting which methods to use.

[6] Williams RM, Myers AM. A new approach to measuring recovery in injured workers with acute low back pain: resumption of activities of daily living scale. Phys Ther 1998; 78:613–623

[7] Kori SH, Miller RP, Todd DD. Kinisophobia: a new view of chronic pain behaviour. Pain Management 1990: 35–43

[8] Waddell G, Newton M, Henderson I, Somerville D, et al. A fear avoidance beliefs questionnaire FABQ and the role of fear avoidance beliefs in chronic low back pain and disability. Pain 1993; 52:157–168

[9] Crombez G, Vlaeyen JWS, Heuts PHTG, Lysens R. Pain-related fear is more disabling than pain itself: evidence on the role of pain related fear in chronic back pain disability. Pain 1999; 80:329–339

[10] Bandura A. Self-efficacy: towards a unifying theory of behaviour change. Psycol Rev 1977; 84:191–215

[11] Harding V, Williams AC de C Williams, Richardson PH, et al. The development of a battery of measures for assessing physical functioning of chronic pain patients. Pain 1994; 58:367–375

[12] Williams RM, Myers AM. Functional abilities confidence scale: a clinical measure for injured workers with acute low back pain. Phys Ther 1998; 78:624–634

[13] Roland M, Morris R. A study of the natural history of low back pain. Part 1. Development of a reliable and sensitive measure of disability in low back pain. Spine 1983; 8:141–144

[14] Bergner M, Bobbitt RA, Carter WB, Gilson BS. The sickness impact profile: development and final revision of a health status measure. Medical Care 1981; 29:787–805

[15] Stratford PW, et al. Defining the minimal level of detectable change for the Roland–Morris questionnaire. Phys Ther 1996; 76:359–368

[16] Mannion AF, Muntener M, Taimela S, Dvorak J. Comparison of three active therapies for chronic low back pain: results of a randomised clinical trial with one year follow-up. Rheumatology 2001; 40:772–778

[17] Morris R, Fairbank J. The Roland-Morris disability questionnaire and the Oswestry disability questionnaire. Spine 2000; 25:3115–3124

[18] Burton AK, Tillotson KM, Main CJ, Hollis S. Psychosocial predictors of outcome in acute and subchronic low back trouble. Spine 1990; 20:722–728

[19] Beurskens AJHM, de Vet HCW, Koke AJA. Responsiveness of functional status in low back pain: a comparison of different instruments. Pain 1996; 65:71–76

[20] Vlaeyen JWS, et al. Fear of movement/reinjury in chronic low back pain and its relation to behavioural performance. Pain 1995; 62:363–372

[21] Turner JA, Jensen MP, Romano JM. Do beliefs, coping and catastrophising independently predict functioning in patients with chronic pain? Pain 2000; 85:115–125

[22] Deyo RA, et al. Outcome measures for studying patients with low back pain. Spine 1994; 19:2032–2036

[23] Peat G. PPA recommendations for low back pain-related functional outcome measures. 2001. CSP website. Ref: CLEF 04

[24] Jensen MP, Romano JM, Turner JA, et al. Patient beliefs predict patient functioning: further support for a cognitive belief model of chronic pain. Pain 1999; 81:95–104

[25] Beaton DE. Understanding the relevance of measured change through studies of responsiveness. Spine 2000; 25:3192–3199

[26] Stratford PW, et al. Defining the minimal level of detectable change for the Roland–Morris questionnaire. Physical Therapy 1996; 76:359–368

[27] Fairbank J, et al. The Oswestry low back pain disability questionnaire. Physiotherapy 1980; 66:271–273

[28] Stratford PW, et al. Development and initial validation of the back pain functional scale. Spine 2000; 25:2095–2102.

[29] Goubert L, Crombez G, Van Damme S, Vlaeyen JWS, Bijttebier P, Roelofs J. Confirmatory factor analysis of the Tampa Scale for Kinesiophobia. Clinical Journal of Pain 2004; 20:103–110.

[30] Vlaeyen JWS, et al. Fear of movement/reinjury in chronic low back pain and its relation to behavioural performance. Pain 1995; 62:363–372

[31] Swinkels-Meewisse EJCM, et al. Psychometric properties of the Tampa scale for Kinesiophobia and the fear avoidance beliefs questionnaire in acute low back pain. Manual Therapy 2003; 8:29–36

[32] Lenthem J, Slade PD, Troup JDG, et al. Outline of a fear avoidance model of exaggerated pain perception. Behavioural Research and Therapy 1983; 21:401–408

[33] Williams RM, Myers AM. Functional abilities confidence scale; a clinical measure for injured workers with acute low back pain. Phys Ther 1998; 78:624–634

[34] Law M, Baptiste S, Mills J. Client centered practice; what does it mean and does it make a difference. Canadian Journal of Occupational Therapy 1995; 62:250–257

[35] Toomey M, Nicholson D, Carswell A. The clinical utility of the Canadian occupational performance measure. Can J Occup Ther 1995; 62:242–249

[36] Ripat J, et al. A comparison of the Canadian occupational performance measure and the health assessment questionnaire. Can J Occup Ther 2001; 68:247–253

[37] McColl MA, et al. Validity and community utility of the Canadian occupational performance measure. Can J Occup Ther 2000; 67:22-30

[38] Walsh DA, et al. Performance in patients with chronic low back pain and the measurement of patient centered outcome. Annual Scientific Meeting of The Pain Society 2003; poster no; 81

[39] Singh S, Morgan M, Scott S, Walters D, Hardman A. Development of a shuttle walking test of disability in patients with chronic airways obstruction. Thorax 1992; 47:1019–1024

[40] Armstrong M, McDonough S, Baxter GD. Reliability and repeatability of the shuttle walk test in chronic low back pain. Physiotherapy 2001; 89

[41] Knox, et al. Reproducibility of walking test results in chronic obstructive airways disease. Thorax 1988; 388–392

[42] Watson PJ, Poulter ME. The development of a functional task-orientated measure of pain behaviour in chronic low back pain patients. Journal of Back and Musculoskeletal Rehabilitation 1997; 9:57–59

[43] Simmonds MJ, Claveau Y. Measures of pain and physical function in patients with low back pain. Physiotherapy Theory and Practice 1997; 13:53–65

[44] Guyatt G, Walter S, Norman G. Measuring change over time; assessing the usefulness of evaluative instruments. Journal of Chronic Disability 1987; 40: 171–178

[45] Linton SJ, Andersson MA. Can chronic disability be prevented? A randomized trial of a cognitive-behavior intervention and two forms of information for patients with spinal pain. Spine 2000; 25:2825-2831

[46] Linton SJ, Ryberg M. A cognitive-behavioral group intervention as prevention for persistent neck and back pain in a non-patient population; a randomized controlled trial. Pain 2001; 90:83–90

Putting it all together

If you only read the books that everyone else is reading, you can only think what everyone else is thinking.

HARUKI MURAKAMI, NORWEGIAN WOOD

INTRODUCTION

Six of the preceding chapters are devoted to mechanisms that create, maintain and modify pain. Only one covers the pain resulting from injury and inflammation, because there are many relevant others. Nevertheless, physical therapy tends to be based on a model that is essentially biomechanical in nature (Fig. 9.1).

Manual therapists tend to approach patients from a mechanical/tissue-based perspective first and only turn to alternative models if this proves to be insufficient. This leads to a number of difficulties for both clinician and patient, as discussed in Chapter 1. On the other hand, the proponents of cognitive-behavioural approaches could be blamed for not paying enough attention to somatic lesions that might respond to manual intervention. In order to make use of the best of physical therapy, psychosocial intervention and neuroscience, clinicians need a new, more inclusive clinical reasoning model (Fig. 9.2).

In Figure 9.2 most space is occupied by the nervous system, in recognition of the fact that pain is a neural phenomenon. The tissues may cause or manifest pain, but it is the nervous system that is responsible for the perception and modification of pain, as well as the response to pain. One reason for depicting the somatic tissues in the perimeter of the diagram is that where pain is concerned they are literally of peripheral importance.

The other reason for representing the somatic tissues as lying on the outside is because they are the most accessible tissues in the body. Receptors at the end of the sensory nerves, sympathetic end organs and end plates in the muscles form interfaces between the somatic tissues and the nervous system. Manual therapy influences the nervous system by affecting the activation of these receptors through the manipulation of the tissues. In addition, it affects cognitive and emotional functions of the brain.

This chapter is devoted to a clinical reasoning process based on this neural model. The aim of the assessment is to get an inventory of all relevant mechanism and the way they interrelate. This informs the

Fig. 9.1 Diagrams representing two conceptual models of musculoskeletal pain. **A.** The traditional musculoskeletal model is based on the arthrokinetic unit of joint and surrounding structures. The factors influencing this unit are of secondary importance. **B.** The biopsychosocial model acknowledges that pain may have a physical component, but focuses on psychological and social influences.

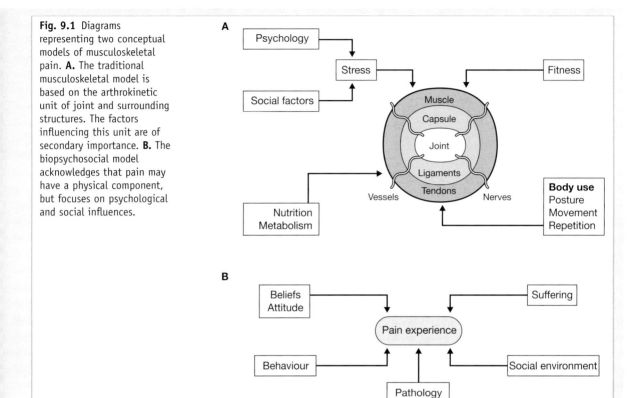

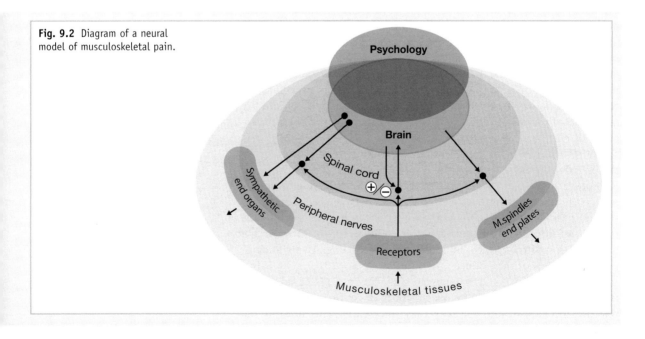

Fig. 9.2 Diagram of a neural model of musculoskeletal pain.

treatment plan, which is designed to address the issues relevant in the individual patient in order of importance.

Principle:

the analysis of all relevant factors improves the chance that treatment will be successful.

THE ASSESSMENT OF MUSCULOSKELETAL PATHOLOGY

Most textbooks for physical therapists outline in great detail how a structure at fault can be found, and how damaged or dysfunctional tissues can be treated. Many therapists follow this course of action, which may well end in frustration if the tissues were not the source of the patient's symptoms or there are additional factors maintaining them. The source of this frustration lies in the underlying assumption that if pain *manifests* in musculoskeletal tissues, it is likely to be *caused* by those tissues. The preceding text makes it clear that this is not justified.

The effective treatment of pain must be based on an assessment procedure and clinical reasoning model that takes into account all factors that may be involved. Clinical reasoning takes the clinician through a process that gradually narrows down the options, until a well-defined hypothesis can be formulated. The difficulty with orthopaedic assessment then, is that the options may be narrowed down too soon, because there is an assumption that the problem is of a musculoskeletal origin. Not considering enough hypotheses is a recognized source of clinical reasoning error.[1]

Much of the art of clinical examination lies in listening to the patient and asking the right questions. By the end of the subjective examination, the clinician should have a fair idea of whether the patient's symptoms point consistently to a musculoskeletal lesion, or whether other factors may be at play (Box 9.1).

Principle:

the musculoskeletal examination is carried out to establish whether the tissues or the pain mechanism need to be treated, or both.

There is a simple change in attitude that can help to safeguard a therapist from frustrating ineffective musculoskeletal treatments. The therapist is advised to ask the question: are there any findings that argue *against* my musculoskeletal hypothesis? This attitude makes the clinician constantly question whether a musculoskeletal diagnosis is certain or even likely (Box 9.2). Pain is a phenomenon of the nervous system, not of the tissues. The mechanocentric model of Figure 1.1 is not appropriate.

Principle:

examination with a view to *ruling out musculoskeletal pathology* increases the chance that pain mechanisms are recognized.

Box 9.1 Problem solving: pain of musculoskeletal origin

What are the characteristics of musculoskeletal pain? Think about the following elements of the assessment procedure:

Description by the patient
1. Aggravating and easing factors tend to be consistent. Rest helps, the affected region is limited.
2. Time course
A: History of injury. Predictable development, in line with healing time.
3. Response to treatment
A: Analgesics and NSAIDs help. Manual treatments and interventions improving posture and movement may be beneficial.
4. Examination findings
A: Consistent response to mechanical tests. No response to distant tests. Selective tissue tensioning applies.
Which descriptions in a patient's history suggests that the patient's pain may not be purely mechanical in origin?
A: Symptom distribution, referred pain. Description of the nature of the pain. Treatment failure (physical and medical). Inconsistent behaviour of symptoms. Effect of non-mechanical influences. Poor patient understanding of the pain and strong emotional response.

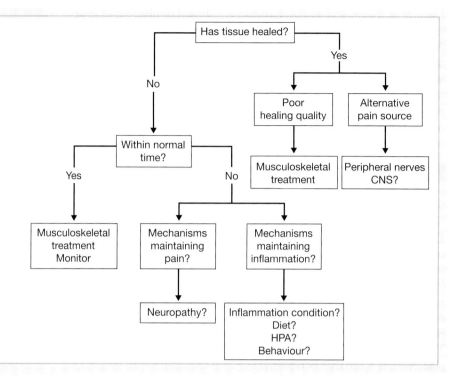

Fig. 9.3 Flowchart of the clinical reasoning model for musculoskeletal pain.

It is possible that there are factors preventing healing. One such factor is the function of the sympathetic and endocrine systems. As discussed in Chapter 5, the former regulates the response of local circulation, while the latter plays a role in determining whether amino acids are available for tissue repair. Other potential factors are the presence of an inflammatory condition such as gout or rheumatoid arthritis or poor diet. Inappropriate behaviour of the patient may also maintain the pathology. Persistent localized pain with musculoskeletal characteristics may be the result of additional neuropathic changes (Box 9.3).

Sub-optimal function of the sympathetic nervous system may be either regional or central. If it is regional, circulation, sweating and pilo-erection may be altered in the affected body part. In addition, organs innervated by the same segments as the affected area may not function optimally (see Ch. 5). Central issues may be related with stress and other psychological issues.

Both sub-optimal sympathetic and endocrine function and inappropriate behaviour warrant investigation of the patient's mindset. This does not mean that the clinician tries to become a psychologist. It is often sufficient to get an idea of the patient's circumstances, as well as their understanding of and emotional reaction to their pain. Inappropriate responses such as overactivity, excessive rest and exercises that are counterproductive are often due to a lack of under-

Box 9.3 Problem solving:neuropathic pain as a masquerader

When a musculoskeletal tissue is injured, peripheral nerves may also be disrupted. How can a therapist decide whether pain that outlasts the healing time is due to ineffective healing mechanisms or neuropathic changes?

A: Description of pain. Allodynia to temperature/touch. Lack of inflammatory signs. Careful sensory testing. Response to analgesics/NSAIDs versus adjuvant drugs.

standing of the pain, fear and anxiety. Furthermore, negative emotions have a direct effect on the hypothalamus–pituitary axis (HPA) and therefore on circulation and metabolism. Only if these issues are addressed does musculoskeletal treatment have a place. However, there may be circumstances where psychological expertise is required, as discussed in Chapter 6.

THE ASSESSMENT OF PAIN PROCESSING STATUS OF THE CENTRAL NERVOUS SYSTEM

The previous section describes how a physical therapist might decide whether their patient's pain is due to nociceptive input from the periphery. Nociceptive input may be the result of tissue damage, inflammation or neuropathic changes. Even if this is thought to be the origin of the pain, the therapist should remain aware that central mechanisms might play a role in maintaining or amplifying symptoms (Fig. 9.4). If the patient has pain in absence of tissue pathology, these mechanisms should feature even more prominently in the clinical reasoning process.

Chapter 4 discusses in detail the model of state dependent processing, which states that the dorsal horn usually passes on its sensory input relatively unchanged. However, under certain circumstances it can either suppress this input or amplify it. When assessing a patient with persistent or poorly understood pain, sensitization of the central nervous system must be considered. The characteristics of this mechanism are presented in Figure 4.8.

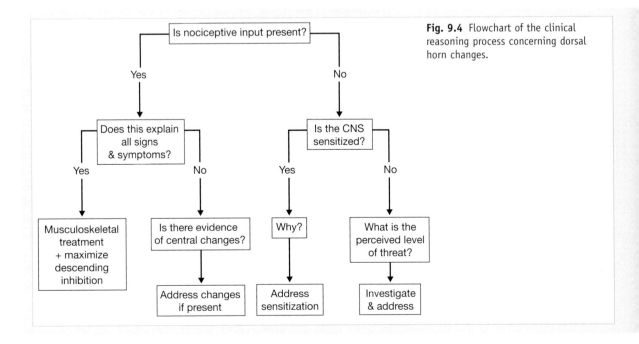

Fig. 9.4 Flowchart of the clinical reasoning process concerning dorsal horn changes.

Box 9.4　Problem solving: allodynia and hyperalgesia

Allodynia is pain as a result of stimulation that normally does not generate pain and hyperalgesia is an enhanced response to painful stimuli. The underlying cause might be a lowered stimulation threshold of peripheral nociceptive nerves (sensitization). On the other hand, allodynia and hyperalgesia may be caused by the dorsal horn's amplification of sensory input.

How does allodynia manifest in patients with musculoskeletal conditions?
A:　As pain in response to the application of gentle mechanical stimuli such as stretch, pressure, massage and palpation. This means that pain may be brought on by certain postures and activities.

Is it necessary to differentiate between the two causes of allodynia and hyperalgesia? Why?
A:　Yes it is, because it is important to use mechanism-based rather than symptom-focused treatments. One cause is the sensitization of peripheral nerves by chemicals released by the tissues. This is treated by helping tissues to heal and inflammation to reduce. The other cause is an alteration in sensory processing in the central nervous system. When this is the underlying mechanism, it is futile to treat the painful tissues alone (Unless done to stimulate specific nerves projecting to the affected spinal cord levels.) Treatment ought to be directed at the processing status of the affected spinal cord levels.

How can a musculoskeletal clinician make this differentiation?
A:　Tissue based pathology has a consistent response to tests, e.g. tests that mechanically load the tissues are uncomfortable, while tests that offload them either ease the discomfort or have no effect on the pain. Symptoms resulting from amplification in the dorsal horn are not necessarily as consistent in their response. Furthermore, central changes are likely to affect other

continued

The dorsal horn receives sensory information from many sources, which is passed on to shared secondary pathways to the brain (Fig. 4.11). Associated with sensitization of the dorsal horn is the concept of reduced selectivity. Normally sensory input from viscera, muscles and skin is kept separate, but when selectivity is low they may influence each other. This means that nociceptive input from one source may be felt as coming from a more superficial tissue. This is known as referred pain. A reduction in selectivity may even lead to a heightened sensitivity of the tissues in which referred pain manifests and this is called referred tenderness.

It is hard to be certain, but with practice the physical therapist can develop skill in deciding whether dorsal horn changes play a role in the patient in the clinic. To summarize, signs and symptoms suggestive of these changes are:

- Tenderness in multiple tissues, especially those with a segmental relationship
- Superficial tenderness
- Referred pain and tenderness
- Allodynia and hyperalgesia.

The therapist who persists in interpreting these findings as signs of damage and inflammation in multiple tissues will find that treatment is extremely likely to result in failure and frustration. As explained above, if the findings indicate a central influence i.e. an influence that is not specific to one tissue, then assessment and treatment should be directed at central and general factors first.

> **Principle:**
>
> the function of the central nervous system must be addressed in the treatment of pain whenever it is found to play a role.

If there are indications that central sensitization may play a role in generating, amplifying or maintaining pain, the clinician may wish to determine which influences cause it to be in this undesirable state. There are two such influences, namely nociceptive input from the body and descending facilitation from the brain (Fig. 9.4). The latter is the subject Assessment of the central scrutinizer below.

If a patient has a neuropathy or a persistent inflammation, this may well fuel changes in sensory processing. The identification of these sources of nociceptive stimulation is relatively straightforward. On the other hand, it is possible that the dorsal horn is being influenced by nociceptive stimulation of the viscera. It is therefore recommended that the therapist ask the patient about the viscera innervated by the same spinal segments as the painful area.

ASSESSMENT OF THE CENTRAL SCRUTINIZER

The brain plays a central role in the perception of and response to pain. It constantly analyses internal and external information and regulates physical processes and behaviour accordingly. It is the brain that decides whether information entering the dorsal horn can safely be suppressed, or whether it needs to be constantly monitored or even amplified. Therefore, if the patient presents with changes suggestive of central sensitization, the assessment should determine whether this is purely a segmental neural change or whether it may be the result of facilitation by the brain.

Facilitation takes place when signals from the body are perceived as relating to a potential threat. Factors that may contribute to the level of threat of a stimulus are:

- *Unfamiliarity.* For example, an experienced athlete is less likely to be disturbed by an injury than a person who is generally inactive or does not have a history of injury. Another example is the patient with a type of pain that they are unfamiliar with, which is common for neuropathic pain.
- *Unpredictability.* If a patient's pain changes for no apparent reason, this may reinforce the brain's vigilance.
- *Indication of physical damage.* Pain is a protective mechanism that demands protective behaviour.
- *Suggestion of impending physical damage.* Part of the protective function of the brain is its capacity to anticipate harmful influences.
- *Mental association with past injuries or threats.* If a person experienced a threatening event in the past, a stimulus that evokes the memory of that event may trigger a strong response. For example, a person who has been hospitalized with a serious lumbar disc prolapse is likely to react strongly to a slight muscle pull in the lower back.
- *Misunderstanding of the nature of the pain.* Poor understanding engenders unpredictability and may lead to the interpretation of pain as a sign of physical damage.

Examples of questions that can give the clinician an indication of the perceived level of threat of a patient's pain are:

- What do you think is causing your pain? This establishes attribution, which is an important factor in determining the brain's response to the pain.
- What explanation have you been given for your pain? Again, this clarifies attribution and its source.
- Do you understand what makes your pain worse or easier? Unpredictability increases the level of threat posed by the pain and enhances the brain's pain response. It is likely to lead to inappropriate coping strategies.
- Have you had a similar pain or injury in the past? This provides insight into familiarity, background and past coping strategies.
- What do you do when you get the pain/when the pain gets worse? Are the patient's coping strategies understandable, helpful, appropriate? Excessive rest is a common unhelpful strategy. While it may alleviate the pain, some of the long-term consequences are loss of

continued

tissues innervated by the same segment(s). Referred pain and trigger points suggest involvement of the dorsal horn.

Suggest treatment strategies for hyperalgesia and allodynia.

A: If tissue based, i.e. primary hyperalgesia, treat the tissues and inflammation. If based on amplification in the dorsal horn, try to alter sensory processing status (see Ch. 4, p. 66). Maximize normal A beta fibre input. Maximize descending inhibition through e.g. explanation and realistic reassurance, advice re helpful strategies, enabling the patient to take up meaningful and enjoyable activities.

Box 9.5 Problem solving: referred pain

How can a clinician distinguish between a local pain and a pain that is referred from a different area?

A: Careful musculoskeletal testing of suspected structures in a way that does not mechanically load the painful area; reproduction of referred pain on testing and palpation of this distant structure; tenderness of more than one structure e.g. skin, muscle, capsule suggests dorsal horn involvement.

How can a clinician differentiate between a referred pain and a pain resulting from a neurogenic problem?

A: Sensory and motor changes absent in referral but possibly present in neurogenic; knowledge of neuro-anatomy and common referral patterns (including trigger points) comparison of tests of musculoskeletal structures that may refer without affecting neuromechanics on the one hand, with tests of neuromechanics that do not affect potential musculoskeletal candidates; using a combined movement type of approach.

Box 9.6 Problem solving: unhelpful beliefs, fear and the brain

A patient interprets pain in the lower back as an indication that the vertebrae are crumbling. It is likely that they are excessively fearful and avoid any activity that creates pain. This is likely to make them unfit, weak and stiff, and therefore less resilient. Therefore, if this belief is not addressed, the patient is not going to benefit from physical therapy. Moreover, they are unlikely to attend at all if the therapy itself causes pain. The therapist may know that it is for the best in the long term, but in the patient's head the alarm bells are ringing with deafening volume!

Box 9.7 Problem solving: functional assessment

A patient would like to return to secretarial work and clean her own house. With the information in Chapter 8, please select functional tests and outcome measures if she has:

- neck pain
- low back pain
- tennis elbow
- arthritic knees.

Think of information that you require about for instance the patient's job, house, beliefs and self-efficacy. Would you be able to get this information from your clinical assessment?

fitness and strength, job loss and reduction in ability to cope with the pain with active strategies.

These questions are not meant to turn the manual therapist into a lay psychologist. Instead, they are asked to provide an insight into the impact of the pain on the patient's pain regulating systems. They also clarify the way the patient interprets the pain.

> *Suggestion:*
> the distance between a patient's self and the pain can be measured in sense of humour. The smaller this distance, the greater the level of threat.

Further insight can be provided by questionnaires such as the Fear Avoidance Beliefs Questionnaire (FABQ) or the Tampa Score of Kinesophobia (Ch. 8). Advantages of these questionnaires are that they enable the clinician to monitor progress objectively and reduce reliance on clinical observation.

THE ASSESSMENT OF FUNCTION

Pain influences function. It motivates behaviours designed to protect and recover. The exact course of action that the brain takes is based on the meaning of the pain. This interpretation is very personal, based on many elements including past experience, explanations and advice from others and the person's psychological makeup. The action that follows from it may be the best choice that the patient could make, but it is not necessarily the most helpful one.

It is not sufficient for therapists to be content with gains in the clinic, if these gains do not translate into the patient's everyday life. A patient who has an improved range of back movement but who feels incapable of taking part in any activity that is important to them, has not made any functional gains. Even if this person's pain has improved, the impact of the pain persists. In the words of Father Claude Larre, a well-known teacher of Chinese thought and medicine:

> If you just treat people in order to relieve their pains, if you are not able to put them back on the right track in accord with the person they are and the situation they are in, then you are only doing half your work, and maybe you are wasting their time not to mention your own.[3]

> *Principle:*
> when assessing function, the therapist tries to think of the patient not as a patient but as a *person*, within his or her own environment.

It is therefore essential that the impact of the pain on the patient's life be assessed (see Ch. 8). Observing the patient at work or at home is a time-consuming process, but the use of questionnaires can provide sufficient insight. In addition, the therapist can use functional tests of activities such as walking or getting up from a chair. When observing the patient perform these tests, it is recommended that the therapist 'switch off' or 'dim' their musculoskeletal-analytical function and try to interpret the quality of movement from a whole body perspective. The following may be helpful:

- Try to imagine what it would be like to move like this. Therapists may wish to re-enact the movement later, in absence of the patient.
- How much use does the patient make of support from for instance a chair, walls or a stick?
- Is the way the patient uses support likely to help their physical problem? If not, what could be the reason for their support seeking behaviour? Try not to jump to conclusions about the patient's sanity or desire for financial compensation. Examples of ineffective use of supports are tubigrip for knee pain or a walking stick used in the wrong hand.
- Is there a discrepancy between the performance level expected on the basis of physical examination and analysis, and that demonstrated by the patient? If there is, it is important that its nature is explored. For example, a patient may have recovered from a back problem from a clinical perspective, but still be terrified of recurrence. This can be reflected in the way they perform or avoid activities. A session of personalized education of pain mechanisms and back pain may address this problem, enabling the patient to return to a high level of function.

Therapists with experience of treating patients with neurological pathologies, for example patients who have had a stroke, will find it easier to interpret function. They can imagine that the patient with pain is having a disturbance of their central nervous system. If there are musculoskeletal pains and dysfunctions, they are seen as consequences of the neurological problems rather than primary. The result of this mental shift is that the therapist looks at issues like quality of movement, functionality and compensatory movements, instead of constantly thinking within a framework of mechanical diagnosis.

TREATMENT

The treatment plan is formulated on the basis of the outcome of the examination and analysis. Patients with persistent pain may have a multitude of symptoms and difficulties, so it is important that the clinician has a clear plan in mind. This plan can be modified in response to the effect of the treatment or lack of it, feedback from the patient and changes in circumstances. In contrast, it is not helpful if the therapist tries everything in their therapeutic repertoire simply to try to resolve the patient's pain.

Rational examination and analysis should lead to a hypothesis, which in turn leads to a treatment strategy. If the treatment results are not forthcoming, the analysis and hypothesis may be revisited. The outcome of this review may be a new hypothesis and/or a new strategy. However, the possibility that effective pain relief is beyond the

Box 9.8 Analysis

The data from the subjective and objective examination are used to form a hypothesis of the mechanisms that create, maintain and alter the patient's pain. As in musculoskeletal diagnosis, the clinician should be able to construct a story of the onset and development of the patient's symptoms. This story should be consistent with the patient's own story and all important examination findings. Inconsistencies suggest an incomplete or incorrect hypothesis, and may warrant further investigation. It must be remembered that malignancy masquerading as musculoskeletal pathology is often discovered because signs and symptoms do not 'add up'.

If the pain is thought to be of musculoskeletal aetiology, the clinician should decide whether it is the lesion that continues to cause the pain. If so, the lesion and its maintaining factors have to be identified and addressed. Both somatic and peripheral neuropathic sources of pain have to be considered. However, even when a lesion can be blamed for the patient's pain, the clinician must be aware that changes in the central nervous system as well as the patient's psychology may need to be addressed.

In many patients with ongoing pain the original lesion, if it was present in the first place, is no longer the main source of the pain. Somehow, the central nervous system continues to behave as if the body were damaged or in danger. Reasons for nociceptive stimulation without obvious injury are the presence of malignancy or systemic pathology. If these factors are absent, the clinician must consider what factors may cause or maintain the activation of pain systems.

Pain related central changes may develop at a spinal level. This can happen purely in response to ongoing nociceptive input from the somatic tissues, but is likely to require the 'go-ahead' from the brain. The decision of the brain to either amplify or suppress pain is based on a host of factors such as homeostasis, cognitions, emotions and higher goals.

continued

continued

At the end of the assessment, the clinician should be able to generate hypotheses based on the following questions:

- What, if anything, is creating nociceptive input into the central nervous system?
- What is determining the response of the central nervous system?

grasp of the clinician must also be considered. The clinician who 'tries everything' is a clinician who does not know what he is doing.

One of the reasons that manual therapists may try treatment after treatment in an attempt to relieve pain, is a lack of knowledge of how pain 'works'. To some extent, an education system that teaches pain physiology as a dry theoretical subject and fails to translate theory in to practice can be blamed for this unfortunate state of affairs. This book is an attempt to remedy this issue. Another reason is the fact that many courses teach *what can be done* with certain techniques, but not what exactly the *boundaries* are. In other words, therapists are taught what they can try but not when to stop trying, or when to not even start.

Knowledge of treatment boundaries tends to develop with experience, but is helped enormously by an incisive clinical reasoning process. Knowing when to stop and why inspires patients with confidence in the clinician and prevents much frustration, both in the patient and the therapist. If a strategy is not worth pursuing, it has to be abandoned in favour of a more effective approach, further investigation or referral to the appropriate professional.

When selecting and evaluating a therapeutic approach, the clinician is advised to be clear whether it is designed to alleviate pain and other symptoms, or to reduce their impact. Therapists often aim for a cure first and only begin to consider pain management approaches when they fail. At this point, the patient is likely to have become disillusioned with the therapeutic process. Even in cases where self-management is highly appropriate, frustration is likely to reduce its chance of success. Once again, this is an argument for the rational analysis of the individual's issues and the formulation of a clear therapeutic strategy.

When making an inventory of the patient's problems, the therapist is advised to estimate the 'relative weight' of each problem, i.e. the magnitude of relevance for the patient's situation and pain. In acute pathologies such as sports injuries, the heaviest issue is the lesion: resolve that and issues such as compensatory movements and psychological stress tend to resolve. However, patients with persistent pain tend to benefit from an approach that considers the central nervous system before turning to the tissues.

> **Principle:**
>
> when formulating a treatment plan, recommended order is as follows:
>
> - Target general issues before specific issues.
> - Target central issues before peripheral issues.

In Figure 9.2 the order of importance is therefore from top to bottom and from centre to periphery. The reason is that central sensitization and altered brain activation can override any potential benefits from a mechanical treatment. In order to treat pain, the therapist has to affect activity in the nervous system. In the injured athlete taking away the noxious stimulus can do this, but in the patient with persistent pain the most important processes are not somatic.

Considering central and general issues first does not imply ignoring the tissues. Even if the therapist decides to follow a pain management approach, he may start with manual techniques to familiarize the patient with sensations of acceptable tissue stretch, or to demonstrate a willingness to help. As long as the therapist is clear that the intervention is part of a strategy designed to affect the central nervous system and mind of the patient, as opposed to the joints and muscles, this is acceptable. It may even be necessary.

The following points are suggested elements in the treatment and management of pain.

Brain intervention: explanation

An explanation of the outcome of the diagnostic process is essential. If the clinician has formed a clear image of how symptoms started and developed, the explanation to the patient is straightforward. It can be used to fill in gaps in the patient's insight and to begin countering unhelpful beliefs. This is also a good time to address uncertainties and unnecessary worries.

The therapist should strive to include the salient points from the patient's own story in the explanation. The successes or failures of self-help strategies and treatments are part of this. If diagnoses were given in the past, both by professionals and lay people, their value should be discussed.

The explanation should include pain physiology as appropriate. Oversimplifications and tissue-based models do not really clarify the unpredictability and sensory qualities of some pain syndrome. Taking time to explain symptoms in the patient's terms, but without talking down to them, is an important tool that should be part of any therapy.

Some of the aims of explanation are: reducing the level of threat and resultant brain activation; empowering the patient by supplying quality information; and forming a strong therapeutic alliance.

Brain intervention: prognosis

The therapist should make clear the available treatment strategies and their potential strengths, limitations and risks. It is up to the patient to make an informed choice, based on the information supplied by the therapist. Explaining the limitations of a technique or strategy reduces frustration if the course of action is abandoned due to a lack of results.

Brain intervention: the introduction of active methods to control pain

Many patients find ways of managing pain that enable them to stay active. A prerequisite for this is that they accept the presence of their pain. Interestingly, this acceptance may open the door to strategies that reduce pain and its impact. On the other hand, a lack of acceptance leads to seeking for a cure. It is the therapist's task to decide and explain whether this search is realistic. If this is outside the therapist's own professional scope, the involvement of a more qualified or experienced professional is invaluable. The temptation to experiment on patients must be resisted.

Relaxation and distraction are strategies that enable patients to cope with ongoing pain by normalizing brain activation and stimulating inhibition of nociceptive processing. However, if there are doubts concerning the diagnosis, for instance if the patient fears an undiscovered tumour, these strategies are likely to cause internal friction that is ultimately counterproductive. The same applies if there is a lack of faith in the therapist's abilities.

It may be helpful to remember that normal physical function is largely unconscious. If a person gets a tin out of the cupboard to make soup, he thinks of the soup and the tin and not of the posture, movement, stretch and strength involved in the process. Pain changes this balance of internal and external focus. One of the aims of treatment can be to normalize it.

Brain intervention: meaningful activities

Engaging in meaningful and enjoyable activities can be a powerful strategy in the management of pain. It can form a distraction from the pain, which is associated with activation of descending inhibition and a reduction in pain-related brain activation. If important activities were lost because of pain and dysfunction and the patient feels unable to formulate or reach new goals in life, they need help with these issues.

If gains in the clinical settings are to be transferred into the patient's life, an exploration of what is important to them is essential. It may be possible to help them to return to activities that were lost, or to find new ways of expressing themselves. What is important is that they are helped to feel like a person rather than a pain. If the patient experiences a gap between themselves and their pain, they can use this gap as the space where they can undertake things.

The more meaning goals and exercises have to a patient, the greater the chance of integration and success. It is important to break down each goal into small, achievable and measurable steps. For example, a person wishing to return to university may have to be able to sit for a maximum of 30 min, carry a brief case of a certain weight over a certain distance, etc. Measurable activities reduce symptom focus and enable objective evaluation of the approach of the goal. They also make possible the estimation of the time required to reach the goal, thereby avoiding seemingly endless and frustrating exercise.

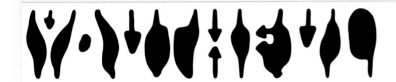

Fig. 9.5 The pain experience: patients tend to focus on their dark experiences, but therapists can make them aware of the remaining positive possibilities. (after [7]).

Donald Price points out that avoidance goals are associated with depression and anxiety when they are not achieved, and relief when they are.[4] This applies to patients who try to find ways to avoid pain. Relief may seem like a positive emotion, but it is only relatively so. On the other hand, approach goals generate feelings of disappointment when not achieved, but excitement and satisfaction when they are. Therefore, the clinician who manages to agree achievable short-term and long-term goals with the patient increases the presence of positive emotions.

Many patients with persistent pain find it hard to think of what they would like to do, because their pains and physical restrictions limit their thinking and imagination. The therapist is in an ideal position to gauge what is possible, and to inspire the patient to revisit their dreams and ambitions. Figure 9.5 shows the black blobs that represent the pains that a patient feels. It is the task of the therapist to make them see the possibilities still open to them.

Some patients may require the help of other agencies, for example in the form of a home assessment by an occupational therapist, help from Social Services, advice from a dietician or careers advice. It is important that therapists communicate effectively with the relevant professionals in order to address barriers to successful management and treatment of pain.

Brain intervention: normalizing cortical representation

Evidence suggests that ongoing pain distorts the representation of the body on the cortex, as discussed in Chapter 7. This may be countered by sensory training regimes such as sensory discrimination training or mirror therapy.[5,6] These therapies can be interpreted as maximizing normal sensory input into the brain, but also as tricking the brain into perceiving the body as appearing and functioning normally.

Brain intervention: create positive expectations

Positive expectations are associated with the release of endorphins in the central nervous system. An optimistic attitude is important, as long as it is tempered by insight into what can realistically be expected from a treatment. However, the therapist should be prepared to be surprised: small miracles do occur and patients may leap forwards unexpectedly, providing learning opportunities for the clinician.

If the patient associates a certain approach with disappointment and other negative emotions, it may be worth avoiding cues linked with this approach. Instead, introduce differences to make it clear to the patient that this therapy is not going to be a re-run of the past.

Dorsal horn intervention: maximizing descending inhibition

Many of the brain interventions discussed above have an effect on descending inhibition and therefore on the way the dorsal horn processes sensory input. Regaining control, understanding, stress reduction and experiencing positive emotions are examples of factors associated with normalization of dorsal horn activity.

Dorsal horn intervention: normalizing sensory input

Activity in the dorsal horn is also regulated by input from the periphery. Normal input is likely to normalize its processing state. It is therefore important to restore normal posture and movement. Stretching exercises, strength training and proprioceptive training can all be used to facilitate normal input into the spinal cord. If a limb is not capable of this, the contralateral limb can be exercised based on a neural overflow principle. If part of the body is affected, the rest of the body may still be exercised to regain fitness. If a movement can be performed properly only within part of the available range or using only part of the maximum strength, the therapist may wish to focus on training within those limits and then gradually expand into the more challenging ranges.

It must be noted that this approach to exercise prescription requires a reconceptualization for some clinicians. The reasons for exercising the body in this way are not based on their benefits for the musculoskeletal tissues. Rather, they are selected because they create A beta fibre input into the spinal segments, while minimizing A delta and C fibre input. Remembering that pain is a phenomenon of the nervous system, which requires treatment that affects the nervous system, may help safeguarding against inappropriate mechanical thinking.

Manual treatments such as massage, myofascial release and Proprioceptive Neuromuscular Facilitation (PNF) can also be adapted to facilitate normal sensory input. However, the effective use of these treatments relies on the patient's understanding that they are part of a transitional phase instead of a way of trying to cure a musculoskeletal pathology.

Dorsal horn intervention: pacing

Wind up is a state in which C fibres discharge for a prolonged period when stimulated. This state requires repeated stimulation for its maintenance, while a lack of nociceptive stimulation extinguishes it. It is possible that this mechanism plays a role in patients with persistent pain, manifesting as prolonged and excessive pain once the patient has exceeded the limits of comfort.

Pacing can be seen as a method that can help a patient to regain activities without reinforcing wind up. In contrast to the healthy athlete, who improves by performing at 100% and then, as it were, forcing a few extra 'percents', the patient with persistent pain needs to follow an approach advocated by more gentle oriental exercise instructors: perform at 70% of your maximum, and then gradually expand that 70%. Neurally, this means that the sensory input generally does not reach nociceptive levels. The mental advantage is that the patient knows that there is a 30% safety margin. Pointing this out to the patient can help to improve relaxation during activity.

At the start, the patient is asked to set baselines by measuring the amount of activity needed to bring on or increase the pain. It is important that the outcome is objectively measurable in distance, steps, time etc., because the patient is then asked to limit activities to 70% of the average maximum. For example, if a patient gets increasing back pain after an average of 10 min of walking, they are asked to never walk for more than 7 min *at a time*. A longer walk is broken down into bouts of 7 min. The patient is encouraged to walk regularly. Many patients have tried to push themselves to walk, resulting in increasing pain and anxiety. Teaching them to pace themselves enables them to walk, get fitter and achieve goals without reinforcing wind up.

Having activity levels that are measurable makes it easier for a patient to comply. Some need an electronic timer that counts down to zero, because they tend to forget to check the time once they have started. Measurement also provides objective feedback about functional activity levels. The latter is also aided by the use of functional outcome measures.

Dorsal horn intervention: segmental therapies

If a patient's pain and/or pathology affect a limited number of spinal segments, treatments designed to affect these segments can be used to normalize dorsal horn function (see Ch. 4). These reflex therapies aim to influence the tissues via the nerves that innervate them. Examples are Connective Tissue Manipulation, cutaneous stimulation to control the bladder and the use of acupuncture points along the spine. It is possible that the release of trigger points can also be a form of reflex therapy.

Peripheral interventions

Interventions aimed at the musculoskeletal tissues are the subject of countless texts on physical therapy. These techniques have very limited usefulness in the management and treatment of pain. However,

APPENDIX 1
Glossary of Pain-related Terminology

Acute pain: pain during tissue damage and healing. For most injuries and conditions, an arbitrary figure of up to 6 weeks tends to be used.

Afferent: a sensory neurone. Primary afferents are nerves taking signals from the tissues to the spinal cord. The signals are transferred to secondary or second order afferents. Finally, tertiary or third order neurones take the signals to the cortex of the brain.

Algogenic: pain causing.

Allodynia: pain resulting from stimulation that is normally innocuous, for example light touch or mild temperature changes. Allodynia may be stimulus specific, for example cold may provoke pain in an area where touch does not.

Anaesthesia dolorosa: pain felt in a numb area.

Analgesia: an absence of pain when a stimulus is applied that is normally perceived as painful.

Causalgia: persistent pain caused by overt damage to a peripheral nerve. This is now classed as Complex Regional Pain Syndrome Type 2.

Central pain: neuropathic pain arising in the central nervous system.

Dysaesthesia: an abnormal sensation that is unpleasant (unlike paraesthesia). When this term is used, it must be specified whether the sensation is felt spontaneously, or whether it is an evoked response.

Efferent: a motor neurone. Strictly speaking, autonomic neurones are efferents because they are part of an output system, but in practice the term efferent is reserved for nerves innervating muscles.

Hyperaesthesia: an increased sensitivity to stimulation. This is a broad term, encompassing both allodynia and hyperalgesia. When only one of these two terms applies, it is preferable to use that term and avoid the term hyperalgesia. As allodynia, it may be stimulus specific.

Hyperalgesia: an increased response to a stimulus that is normally painful. The pain is stronger than it would normally be.

Hyperpathia: an abnormally painful reaction to a stimulus, as well as an increased threshold. This may involve a change in the subject's perception of the nature and location of the stimulus. The stimulus may be felt in an area away from the actual site of stimulation, or it may radiate away from that site. Sensation may persist once stimulation has ceased. The pain is often described as explosive in nature.

Hypoaesthesia: a reduced sensitivity to stimulation. This is the opposite of hyperaesthesia. Again, it is stimulus specific.

Neurogenic pain: pain originating from within the nervous system itself, either because of a lesion or a neural dysfunction. Neurogenic pain can be peripheral or central in origin, or both.

Neuropathic pain: often used as synonymous with the term neurogenic pain. The term neuropathic may be reserved for more persistent neurogenic pains.

Nociception: sensation as a result of the stimulation of nociceptive nerves. Although this stimulation commonly causes pain, it may not. Furthermore, pain may exist in absence of nociception.

Nociceptive nerves: relatively thin afferents of type C and A delta.

Nociceptor: a receptor preferentially sensitive to inflammation, tissue damage and stimuli that could cause damage if prolonged or progressed. Nociceptors are found at the end of nociceptive nerves.

Pain (IASP definition[1]): an unpleasant sensory and emotional experience associated with actual or potential tissue damage, or described in terms of such damage. Note: pain is not unpleasant to everyone under all circumstances. It is a highly subjective experience.

Pain threshold: the lowest level of stimulation that is experienced as pain by a subject. It must be realized that this is specific not only for the individual, but also for the type of stimulus and the context. The pain threshold is highly variable between individuals, as well as within the individual. It is meaningless to say that someone has a high pain threshold, because it is not an absolute measure.

Pain tolerance level: the greatest level of pain a subject is willing to tolerate. As with pain threshold, this is a highly individual measure, dependent on context and type of stimulus.

Paraesthesia: an abnormal sensation that is not unpleasant. In practice, this includes sensations of pins and needles or ants crawling on the skin.

Persistent or chronic pain: pain outlasting the time in which completion of the healing process is expected. The arbitrary figure of more than 3 months tends to be used. The term may also be used for ongoing pain not caused by a lesion. Many patients refer to pain that is intense as chronic, so the term persistent pain may be less ambiguous.

Segment: an innervation level of the spinal cord, for instance L3 or T9. Each spinal nerve contains nerve fibres from one single segment.

Segmental therapy: treatment aimed at influencing the function of the nerves of a spinal segment, usually in order to affect a change in tissues or organs innervated by that segment.

Somatic sensation: sensation provided by receptors in the body.[2] This term most commonly refers to sensation of the skin and musculoskeletal system. When the term somatic is used for efferent nerves, it refers to motor neurones as opposed to autonomic nerves.

Subacute pain: pain experienced while the healing process is resolving. The arbitrary figure of six to twelve weeks tends to be used.

References

[1] International Association for the Study of Pain. IASP pain terminology. Available online: www.iasp-pain.org/terms-p.html 18-12-2003

[2] Gardner E, Martin J, Jessell T. The bodily senses. In: Kandel E, Schwartz J, Jessell T, eds. Principles of neural science. New York: McGraw-Hill, 2000: 430–450

APPENDIX 2
Roland Morris Disability Questionnaire[1]

When you have pain you may find it difficult to do some of the things you normally do. This list contains some sentences that people have used to describe themselves when they have pain. When you read them you may find that some of them describe you very well as you are today. As you read the list, think of yourself today. When you read a sentence that describes you today, put a {√} against it. If the sentence does not describe you then leave the box blank and go on to the next one. Remember, only tick the sentence if you are sure that it describes you today.

1. I stay at home most of the time because of my pain ❏
2. I change positions more frequently to try to get my pain comfortable ❏
3. I walk more slowly than usual because of my pain ❏
4. Because of my pain I am not doing any of the jobs I usually do around the house ❏
5. Because of my pain, I use a handrail to get up stairs ❏
6. Because of my pain, I lie down to rest more often ❏
7. Because of my pain, I have to hold onto something to get out of an easy chair ❏
8. Because of my pain I try to get other people to do things for me ❏
9. I get dressed more slowly than usual because of my pain ❏
10. I only stand up for short periods of time because of my pain ❏
11. Because of my pain, I try not to bend or kneel down ❏
12. I find it difficult to get out of my chair because of my pain ❏
13. I am in pain almost all of the time ❏
14. I find it difficult to turn over in bed because of my pain ❏
15. My appetite is not very good because of my pain ❏
16. I have trouble putting on my shoes (or stockings) because of my pain ❏
17. I only walk short distances because of my pain ❏
18. I sleep less well because of my pain ❏
19. Because of my pain, I get dressed with help from somebody else ❏
20. I sit down most of the day because of my pain ❏
21. I avoid heavy jobs around the house because of my pain ❏
22. Because of my pain, I am more irritable and bad tempered with people than usual ❏
23. Because of my pain, I go upstairs more slowly than usual ❏
24. I stay in bed most of the time because of my pain. ❏

Reference

[1] Roland M, Fairbank J. The Roland Morris disability questionnaire and the Oswestry disability questionnaire. *Spine* 2000; 25:3115–3124

APPENDIX 3
Owestry Disability Questionnaire[1]

Please complete this questionnaire. It is designed to give us information as to how your back (or leg) trouble has affected your ability to manage in everyday life. Please answer every section. Mark one box only in each section that most closely describes you today.

SECTION 1: Pain Intensity
- ❏ I have no pain at the moment
- ❏ The pain is very mild at the moment
- ❏ The pain is moderate at the moment
- ❏ The pain is fairly severe at the moment
- ❏ The pain is very severe at the moment
- ❏ The pain is the worst imaginable at the moment

SECTION 2: Personal Care (Washing, Dressing, etc.)
- ❏ I can look after myself normally without causing extra pain
- ❏ I can look after myself normally but it causes extra pain
- ❏ It is painful to look after myself and I am slow and careful
- ❏ I need some help but can manage most of my personal care
- ❏ I need help every day in most aspects of personal care
- ❏ I do not get dressed, wash with difficulty and stay in bed

SECTION 3: Lifting
- ❏ I can lift heavy weights without extra pain
- ❏ I can lift heavy weights but it causes me extra pain
- ❏ Pain prevents me lifting heavy weights off the floor but I can manage if they are conveniently placed e.g. on a table
- ❏ Pain prevents me lifting heavy weights but I can manage light to medium weights if they are conveniently positioned
- ❏ I can only lift very light weights
- ❏ I cannot lift or carry anything

SECTION 4: Walking
- ❏ Pain does not prevent me walking any distance
- ❏ Pain does not prevent me walking more than 2 kilometres
- ❏ Pain prevents me from walking more than 1 kilometre
- ❏ Pain prevents me walking more than 500 metres
- ❏ I can only walk using a stick or crutches
- ❏ I am in bed most of the time

SECTION 5: Sitting
- ❏ I can sit in any chair as long as I like
- ❏ I can only sit in my favourite chair as long as I like
- ❏ Pain prevents me sitting for more than one hour
- ❏ Pain prevents me sitting for more than 30 minutes
- ❏ Pain prevents me sitting for more than 10 minutes
- ❏ Pain prevents me sitting at all

SECTION: Standing
- ❏ I can stand as long as I want without extra pain
- ❏ I can stand as long as I want but it gives me extra pain
- ❏ Pain prevents me from standing for more than 1 hour
- ❏ Pain prevents me from standing for more than 30 minutes
- ❏ Pain prevents me from standing for more than 10 minutes
- ❏ Pain prevents me from standing at all

SECTION 7: Sleeping
- ❏ My sleep is never disturbed by pain
- ❏ My sleep is occasionally disturbed by pain
- ❏ Because of pain I have less than 6 hours sleep
- ❏ Because of pain I have less than 4 hours sleep
- ❏ Because of pain I have less than 2 hours sleep
- ❏ Pain prevents me from sleeping at all

Section 8: Sex Life (if applicable)
- ❏ My sex life is normal and causes no extra pain
- ❏ My sex life is normal but causes some extra pain

❏ My sex life is nearly normal but is very painful
❏ My sex life is severely restricted by pain
❏ My sex life is nearly absent because of pain
❏ Pain prevents any sex life at all

Section 9: Social Life

❏ My social life is normal and gives me no extra pain
❏ My social life is normal but increases the degree of pain
❏ Pain has no significant effect on my social life apart from limiting my more energetic interests e.g. sport
❏ Pain has restricted my social life and I do not go out as often
❏ Pain has restricted my social life to my home
❏ I have no social life because of pain

Section 10: Travelling

❏ I can travel anywhere without pain
❏ I can travel anywhere but it gives me extra pain
❏ Pain is bad but I manage journeys over 2 hours
❏ Pain restricts me to journeys of less than 1 hour
❏ Pain restricts me to journeys under 30 minutes
❏ Pain prevents me from travelling except to receive treatment

score: /   x 100 =   %

Scoring: For each section the total possible score is 5: if the first statement is marked the section score = 0, if the last statement is marked it = 5.

If all ten sections are completed the score is calculated as follows:

Example: 16 (total scored)
             50 (total possible score) x 100 ≥ 32%

If one section is missed or not applicable the score is calculated:

             16 (total scored)
             45 (total possible score) x 100 = 35.5%

Minimum Detectable Change (90% confidence): 10.5% points (change of less than this may be attributable to error in the measurement).

Reference

[1] Roland M, Fairbank J. The Roland Morris disability questionnaire and the Oswestry disability questionnaire. Spine 2000; 25:3115–3124

APPENDIX 4
Back Pain Functional Scale

On the questions listed below we are interested in knowing whether you are having **ANY DIFFICULTY** at all with the activities **because of your back problem** for which you are currently seeking attention.
Please provide an answer for each activity.

Today, do you or <u>would you have</u> any DIFFICULTY at all with the following activities BECAUSE OF YOUR BACK PROBLEM?

Circle one number on each line:
Unable to perform activity (0)   Extreme Difficulty (1)   Quite a bit of Difficulty (2)   Moderate Difficulty (3)
A Little bit of Difficulty (4)   No Difficulty (5)

1. Any of your usual work, housework, or school activities	0 1 2 3 4 5
2. Your usual hobbies, recreational, or sporting activities	0 1 2 3 4 5
3. Performing heavy activities around your home	0 1 2 3 4 5
4. Bending or stooping	0 1 2 3 4 5
5. Putting on your shoes or socks (pantyhose)	0 1 2 3 4 5
6. Lifting a box of groceries from the floor	0 1 2 3 4 5
7. Sleeping	0 1 2 3 4 5
8. Standing for 1 hour	0 1 2 3 4 5
9. Walking a mile	0 1 2 3 4 5
10. Going up or down 2 flights of stairs (about 20 stairs)	0 1 2 3 4 5
11. Sitting for 1 hour	0 1 2 3 4 5
12. Driving for 1 hour	0 1 2 3 4 5

SUBTOTALS

TOTAL SCORE =   /60

Permission obtained from author (Paul Stratford) and publisher (J.Rheumatology).[1]

Reference

[1] Stratford PW, Binkley JM. A comparison study of the Back Pain Functional Scale and the Roland Morris questionnaire. Jnl Rheum. 2000; 27:1928–1936

APPENDIX 5
The Tampa Scale, Miller, Kori and Todd 1991

Read each question and circle the number that best corresponds to how *you* feel.

Strongly disagree (1)   somewhat disagree (2)   somewhat agree (3)   strongly agree (4)

1. I'm afraid that I might injure myself again if I exercise	1 2 3 4
2. If I were to try to overcome it my pain would increase	1 2 3 4
3. My body is telling me I have something dangerously wrong	1 2 3 4
4. People aren't taking my medical condition seriously enough	1 2 3 4
5. My accident has put my body at risk for the rest of my life	1 2 3 4
6. Pain always means I have injured my body	1 2 3 4
7. I am afraid I might injure myself accidentally	1 2 3 4
8. Simply being careful that I do not make any unnecessary movements is the safest thing I can do to prevent my pain from worsening	1 2 3 4
9. I wouldn't have this amount of pain if there weren't something potentially dangerous going on in my body	1 2 3 4
10. Pain lets me know when to stop exercising so I don't injure myself	1 2 3 4
11. It's really not safe for a person with a condition like mine to be physically active	1 2 3 4
12. I can't do all the things normal people do because it's too easy for me to get injured	1 2 3 4
13. No one should have to exercise when she/he is in pain	1 2 3 4

Thank you for taking the time to answer these questions

Reproduced with permission from [1] and the International Association for the Study of Pain.

Reference

[1] Vlaeyen JWS, Kole-Snijders AM, Boeren RG, van Eek H. Fear of movement/(re)injury in chronic low back pain and its relation to behavioural performance. Pain 1995; 62:363–372

APPENDIX 6
Fear Avoidance Beliefs Questionnaire[1]

Here are some of the things which other patients have told us about their pain. For each statement please circle any number from 0–6 to say how much physical activities such as bending, lifting, walking or driving would affect *your* back pain.

Completely disagree?   Unsure?   Completely agree?

1. My pain was caused by physical activity   0 1 2 3 4 5 6

2. Physical activity makes my pain worse   0 1 2 3 4 5 6

3. Physical activity might harm my back   0 1 2 3 4 5 6

4. I should not do physical activities that (might) make my pain worse   0 1 2 3 4 5 6

5. I cannot do physical activities which (might) make my pain worse   0 1 2 3 4 5 6

The following statements are about how your normal work affects or would affect your back pain.
Completely disagree?   Unsure?   Completely agree?

1. My pain was caused by my work or by an accident at work   0 1 2 3 4 5 6

2. My work aggravated my pain   0 1 2 3 4 5 6

3. I have a claim for compensation for my pain   0 1 2 3 4 5 6

4. My work is too heavy for me   0 1 2 3 4 5 6

5. My work makes or would make my pain worse   0 1 2 3 4 5 6

6. My work might harm my back   0 1 2 3 4 5 6

7. I should not do my normal work with my present pain   0 1 2 3 4 5 6

8. I cannot do my normal work with my present pain   0 1 2 3 4 5 6

9. I cannot do my normal work till my pain is treated   0 1 2 3 4 5 6

10. I do not think I will be back to my normal work within 3 months   0 1 2 3 4 5 6

11. I do not think I will ever be able to go back to that work   0 1 2 3 4 5 6

Scoring Scale 1: fear-avoidance beliefs about work – items 6, 7, 9, 10, 11, 12, 15
           Scale 2: fear-avoidance beliefs about physical activity – items 2, 3, 4, 5.
Reproduced with permission from [1] and the International Association for the Study of Pain

Reference

[1] Waddell G, Newton M, Henderson I, Somerville D, Main CJ. A fear avoidance beliefs questionnaire (FABQ) and the role of fear avoidance beliefs in chronic low back pain and disability. Pain 1993; 52:157–168

APPENDIX 7
Addresses and websites

Chartered Society of Physiotherapy
14 Bedford Row
London WC1R 4ED
UK
Tel: + 44 (0) 20 7242 1941
www.csp.org.uk
Contains review of outcome measures

International Association for the Study of Pain
909 NE 43rd Street
Suite 306
Seattle
WA 98105-6020
USA
Tel: + 1 206 547 6409
www.iasp-pain.org
Contains a glossary of pain terms

Pain Concern
PO Box 13256
Haddington
EH41 4YD
UK
Tel: +44 (0) 1620 822 572
www.painconcern.org.uk
Contains advice leaflets that can be ordered

Physiotherapy Pain Association
Kestrel
Swanpool, Falmouth
Cornwall TR11 5BD
UK
www.ppaonline.co.uk
Contains downloadable documents for clinicians and a
  lively discussion page

***Stop Pain* (Beth Israel Medical Centre)**
www.stoppain.org
Contains downloadable PowerPoint presentations and
  information for professionals

Electrotherapy website by Tim Watson
www.electrotherapy.org/Electro/healing/tissue.htm
Contains tissue healing and the effects of electrotherapy

Chronic Pain
A well made and useful CD with patient guidance and
  guided relaxation can be ordered from the website or
  by sending a cheque for £4.50 to Pain CD, PO Box 84,
  Blackburn BB2 7GH, UK
www.chronicpain.org.uk

The British Pain Society
21 Portland Place
London W1B 1PY
UK
www.britishpainsociety.org
Contains downloadable pain scale in many languages

Index